Multiple Sclerosis

The Guide to Treatment and Management

Sixth Edition

Chris H. Polman, MD, PhD
Professor of Neurology
Free University Medical Centre
Amsterdam, The Netherlands

Alan J. Thompson, MD, FRCP, FRCPI
Garfield Weston Professor of Clinical Neurology and Neurorehabilitation
Institute of Neurology, University College London
Clinical Director, National Hospital for Neurology and Neurosurgery
London, England

T. Jock Murray, OC, MD, FRCPC, MACP, FRCP
Professor of Medicine (Neurology)
Professor of Medical Humanities
Dalhousie University
Halifax, Nova Scotia, Canada

Allen C. Bowling, MD, PhD
Medical Director
Rocky Mountain Multiple Sclerosis Center
Englewood, Colorado, USA
Clinical Associate Professor of Neurology
University of Colorado Health Sciences Center
Denver, Colorado, USA

John H. Noseworthy, MD, FRCPC
Professor and Chair
Department of Neurology
Mayo Clinic College of Medicine
Rochester, Minnesota, USA

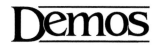

Demos Medical Publishing, LLC, 386 Park Avenue South, New York, New York 10016

Visit our website at www.demosmedpub.com

Library of Congress Cataloging-in-Publication Data

Multiple sclerosis : the guide to treatment and management / Chris H. Polman . . . [et al.].—6th ed.
    p. cm.
    Includes bibliographical references and index.
    ISBN 1-932603-51-4 (alk. paper)
  1. Multiple sclerosis.   2. Multiple sclerosis—Treatment.
  I. Polman, Chris.
  RC377.5583   2006
  616.8'3406—dc22

                                  2005018980

Printed in Canada

Multiple Sclerosis

The Guide to Treatment and Management

Sixth Edition

Contents

Foreword

Information about multiple sclerosis (MS) has never been more widely available. The Internet has enabled people affected by MS and health professionals in every part of the world to share their knowledge about effective treatments and has created a real opportunity for truly international cooperation in finding a cure and ending the devastating effects of this disease.

However, this rich source of facts, advice, and support is tempered by misinformation and opinion that has also been disseminated. Therefore it becomes increasingly important to deliver up-to-date and accurate information in order to distinguish valid treatments from those that are ineffective or even dangerous.

The Multiple Sclerosis International Federation (MSIF) prides itself on providing quality information on all aspects of MS, and is particularly pleased to sponsor this sixth edition of *Multiple Sclerosis: The Guide to Treatment and Management.* It is the result of meticulous work by the International Medical and Scientific Board of the MSIF to establish authoritative guidance on a wide range of therapies currently being used in the management of MS. The book has been completely revised to reflect the latest available information about this disease.

People with MS, their friends and caregivers, and health care professionals, will find great value in the Guide, and the MSIF thanks everyone who has contributed so generously of their time to produce this edition.

Christine Purdy
Chief Executive
Multiple Sclerosis International Federation
June 2005

Preface

Since publication of the fifth edition of *Multiple Sclerosis: The Guide to Treatment and Management* in 2001, the ability to better understand relevant disease mechanisms as well as to modify the course of the disease has had a profound impact on the outlook of people with multiple sclerosis (MS). There are more grounds for hope now than four years ago, although we must also recognize that in our attempts to advance the art of medicine unexpected complications can occur.

Improvements have also been achieved in symptomatic management and neurologic rehabilitation. New drugs have been developed, and more effective ways of administering older drugs devised. Controlled trials of certain aspects of neurorehabilitation have shown that there are many effective approaches to management of MS.

This book provides a comprehensive, readily accessible guide to the wide diversity of therapeutic options now available to treat MS. As with previous editions, all therapies in current use are discussed in detail and a statement given for each that reflects consensus opinion about each therapy's usefulness and effectiveness.

In deciding whether to adopt a particular form of treatment (whether it be medical, surgical, rehabilitative, or "alternative"), it is necessary to weigh the evidence about its effectiveness and the risk and nature of side effects for the individual patient. We have done that in this book to the best of our ability, trying to provide a general recommendation. Wherever possible we have

based our recommendations on scientific, peer-reviewed pub-
lications.

Readers of the previous editions will notice that we have
added a guide to further reading for additional details about
particular treatments and how their effectiveness and side effects
have been assessed. Summaries or abstracts of the journal articles
cited in this book may be found through "Medline" searches,
available through the website of the National Library of Medicine
(www.hlm.nih.gov); entire articles may be obtained from medical libraries.

As today the Internet is the first place to which many people
turn for information the contents of this book are available on
the Multiple Sclerosis International Federation (MSIF) Web site,
"The World of MS" (www.msif.org). The online version allows
for rapid updating of material between print editions, and we
urge readers to use this resource to access newly available
information.

All material included in this volume was reviewed by members of the International Medical & Scientific Board (IMSB) of
MSIF, all of whom are neurologists in active practice who treat
patients with MS on a daily basis; the authors thank them for
their many suggestions and comments. Their opinions are based
not only on published data but also on their daily experiences
and information from trusted colleagues. We give special thanks
to the Multiple Sclerosis International Federation, the official
sponsor of this volume, for facilitating publication of this
sixth edition.

The MSIF International Medical and Scientific Board (IMSB) Medical Management Committee

Dr. Fernando Cáceres
Clínica de Neuroimmunología
División Neurología
Hospital Ramos Mejía
Buenos Aires, Argentina

Professor Michel Clanet
Hôpital Purpan
Toulouse, France

Professor Hans-Peter Hartung
Department of Neurology
Karl-Franzens-Universität
  Graz
Graz, Austria

Professor Jürg Kesselring
Department of Neurology
Rehabilitation Center
Valens, Switzerland

Dr. Elizabeth McDonald
Multiple Sclerosis Society
Victoria, Australia

Dr. Xavier Montalban
Neurology Department
H.G.U. Vall D'Hebron
Barcelona, Spain

Dr. John Noseworthy
Department of Neurology
Mayo Clinic College of
  Medicine
Rochester, Minnesota

Dr. Chris H. Polman
Department of Neurology
Free University Medical
  Centre
Amsterdam, The Netherlands

Dr. Carlo Pozzilli
Department of Neurological
  Sciences
University of Rome
Rome, Italy

Dr. Juhani Ruutiainen
Masku Neurological
  Rehabilitation Centre
Masku, Finland

Dr. Randall T. Schapiro
Department of Neurology
University of Minnesota
Minneapolis, Minnesota

Professor Alan J. Thompson
Institute of Neurology
University College
London, England

Chapter 1

Introduction: The Changing Understanding of MS

There is a good reason why this book is being continuously revised: The research and information on how best to treat and manage persons with multiple sclerosis (MS) is rapidly changing and advancing.

Jean Martin Charcot described the clinical and pathological features of MS in 1868, and for the next century there was an understanding of the nature of the disease according to the clinical and laboratory methods of the day. It was believed to be a disease primarily affecting young adults that began with an attack of neurological symptoms. A number of attacks might occur, and these were noted to be related to scattered inflammatory lesions (plaques) in the white matter of the central nervous system (CNS). The inflammatory lesions were characterized by a breakdown of the myelin that surrounds the central axon of the nerves, but with relative preservation of the axons. After a long period when there were frequent attacks and remissions of symptoms, there was often a stage of slow progression of neurological deficit. This picture seemed to fit what physicians were seeing in most patients. However, in the last few years there has been a rapid expansion of the research effort to better understand the disease and its underlying mechanisms. This new information has provided a different understanding of the disease.

We now see that MS does not start with the first attack, because there is information that there has been disease activity long before this, probably many years before. Although it mostly affects young adults, it can also occur in children or much older adults. Patches of inflammation and demyelination certainly are present in the white matter of the CNS, and can be seen on magnetic resonance imaging (MRI), but there is increasing evidence that the changes in the disease are much more widespread than the scattered lesions would suggest, including in areas previously thought to be normal. The information from serial MRI studies also shows that there is a process of ongoing activity, even when the person does not notice any new symptoms. For over a century the focus has been on the breakdown of the myelin sheath that surrounds the central axon of the nerve, but current interest centers on the axon and on the demonstration that there is subtle but important and widespread axonal change. This widespread axonal damage may be more important in causing the progression seen later in the disease. Although always regarded as a white matter disease, there is now evidence that changes may occur in the grey matter as well. From this brief outline it is clear that understanding of the underlying processes in MS is rapidly changing, and these clarified concepts are crucial in the development of new therapies and treatment approaches for persons with MS.

There is also substantial new information about the genetic aspect of the disease, as well as the potential "triggers" that might precipitate the appearance of the disease in someone who is predisposed to the disorder. The complex immunological changes that affect the myelin and axons are becoming better understood, allowing the development of therapies that are focused on specific steps and pathways in the immune system.

It has long been noted that MS has a variable incidence in different parts of the world, and epidemiology research reveals possibilities for why some populations are more at risk than others. Studies of the natural history of the disease clarify the various patterns of MS that can occur. Using this natural history information, investigators will be able to better measure whether new therapies will alter the eventual outcome of the disease.

Almost all of the major advances in medicine have occurred in a steady, stepwise fashion, with new information and advances from basic research giving insights leading to the next stage. Subsequent research has led to other stages prior to the eventual "discovery." Although patients and physicians are naturally waiting impatiently for major advances, the pace of change and advance is proceeding at an unparalleled rate, and the view is more hopeful than ever.

BETTER DIAGNOSIS

Diagnosis of MS has always been a clinical decision, but many tests and criteria have assisted the clinician in arriving at conclusions. Tests such as MRI, the examination of the cerebrospinal fluid (CSF), and visual evoked potentials (VEP) are helpful in confirming the clinical suspicion of MS.

The clinician first conducts a history of the features of the patient's story of neurological symptoms, and then a neurological examination to assess how the nervous system has been affected. Defined criteria are used to conclude whether the features fulfill the clinical diagnosis. Tests then help confirm the suspicion that the disease is or is not present. Having defined criteria for the clinical diagnosis and criteria for a positive MRI for MS allow for more precision in the diagnosis and lessen the likelihood of a premature diagnosis in questionable cases wherein the MS-like symptoms may be due to some other condition. Just as with other aspects of the disease, we learn more as the criteria are adjusted and improved. The McDonald Criteria are currently being used to incorporate the clinical understanding. Helpful tests such as MRI, CSF examination, and visual evoked potentials are also used.

Although the MRI is a relatively new test in the last few decades, it is of great diagnostic assistance to the clinician. It is valuable in revealing much about the activity of the disease, helpful in assessing potentially effective drugs, and useful as part of the evaluation of the impact of new therapies.

As we become aware of the variety of presentations and courses of MS, we are able to diagnose cases that would have been undiagnosed in the past, or would have gone on for many years without a diagnosis.

THERAPY THAT IS MORE FOCUSED

The current approaches to therapy are becoming much more focused on the specific mechanisms thought to be important in the disease, as research teaches more about the complex phenomena involved in the disease.

It was noted by the earliest observers of MS that inflammatory lesions caused local patches of demyelination. When corticosteroids were discovered, their remarkable antiinflammatory activity was used in MS for acute attacks of the disease. It is now clear that steroids in high doses, usually given intravenously, can reduce inflammation and shorten the attack of symptoms, but they probably do not have more than a short-term benefit. Early observers realized that something more than a drug to reduce inflammation was necessary. When it became clear that an immunological reaction was how the demyelination occurred, general agents that could stimulate or suppress the immune system were tried, but they also had little effect and had many side effects. Over the years the complexity of the immune reaction was better understood, and now agents that target various steps are being developed and tested. This explains why so much basic research needs to be done before an effective drug is available. It is possible, but less likely, that very effective therapy will become available *before* we understand the disease better through basic research into the amazing ways the nervous system reacts, responds, heals, and fails under the influences of disease. There is an increasing sense of hope in patients, their physicians, and researchers, because of the research effort and the number of studies, and because the community of investigators has never been so great and it increases each year.

Since the 1970s, neurologists have been able to modify the acute attacks of the disease, but they have also searched for agents that would modify the eventual outcome of MS. In the last two decades a number of agents have been tested, and for the first time show evidence that they can modify the number and severity of the attacks of MS and reduce the activity seen on MRI. We would expect this modification of the inflammatory activity of the disease to reduce the rate of eventual progression of the disease, but better long-term studies will be necessary to convincingly demonstrate this most important outcome effect.

An exciting development has been the observation that there are at least four patterns of reaction involved in the areas of myelin and axon damage. This may lead to different focused therapeutic interventions, depending on the pattern of neurological damage, but will involve finding practical ways to identify the patterns in a patient, especially early in the disease.

The challenges are great, but there is hope that in the over one hundred clinical trials, the over thirty different agents being studied, and the fourteen combination studies being conducted that substantial benefits will continue to come to the many who currently suffer from MS.

EVIDENCE OF EFFECTIVENESS IN THERAPY OF MS

For centuries, therapies have been applied by trial and error, and varied according to the theory of disease at the time. The main measure of effectiveness has been the experience of the practitioner. But theories can be incorrect and experience faulty. The fact that something has been used for many years, even for centuries, is not assurance that it is helpful. The best example is bleeding, which was a mainstay of therapy for most of the serious diseases for thousands of years, even though we now know it was probably more harmful than helpful.

Confidence that something is helpful in the treatment of MS requires evidence, and there are different levels of evidence. A neighbor's claim that a particular medicine helped her or a story of someone who responded dramatically to a therapy (*anecdotal evidence*) constitutes weak evidence. More people claiming the same thing adds weight, but is still not solid evidence, since almost any approach – useful or useless – has enthusiastic believers.

Stronger evidence would be provided by a carefully followed group of patients in an *open trial* – but since both the patient and physician are aware of the nature of the therapy, the results can be affected by bias and by the placebo effect. In addition, in an open trial patients may drop out if they do not do well or feel worse, so the therapist accumulates all the good responders and has the impression that most of the treated patients do well.

Defining how patients will be treated and assessed over a future period – a *prospective trial* – is stronger evidence than a study that looks back in time to see how people fared from a treatment – a *retrospective trial.*

Monumental advances have been made in the last half century in the development of a scientific approach to measurement of *effectiveness versus risk* for a therapy. The most obvious is the development of the *double-blind, placebo-controlled, randomized, clinical trial* (RCT). The randomized clinical trial can be used to study new drugs, but also surgical procedures and other methods of care.

Trials can be made stronger by using a *placebo control group* to compare with the group on the proposed therapy. The two groups are *matched* for as many factors as possible (similar age, sex, duration, type, and severity of disease, and any other factors that seem important), and by keeping the therapist and the patient *blinded* as to whether they are receiving the treatment or the placebo. Only an overseeing *safety committee* is able to access information as to what patients are taking in the trial.

Many alleged treatments can be put forward as beneficial for patients with MS, but it is humbling to realize that what seems like a good idea may not be helpful, and may even be harmful. Some approaches may seem to be helpful because we want them to be, and we take any sign of improvement to be due to the treatment. We are realizing that no matter how objective we may try to be, our biases and our hopes influence what we think we are seeing. Clinical trials are designed to reduce *bias* as much as possible.

When using a therapy, the benefit seen may be due to the *placebo effect*, which is a real effect that has been shown to be significant in therapies used for MS. The interesting and complex nature of the placebo effect is now better understood, and the design of clinical trials allows for assessment of a study drug in comparison to the effect one might see with a placebo.

Clinical trials also use statistical methods to indicate how many patients need to be studied in equal groups and for how long, in order to demonstrate a significant effect if there is one. The process of *randomization* of patients assures that the groups to be compared, one on the study drug and the other on a similar appearing placebo, are similar on defined characteristics.

In recent years, a technique called *meta-analysis* has added even stronger evidence about therapies. Meta-analysis takes all of the well designed trials that meet defined criteria and analyses their results in order to reach a conclusion about the safety and effectiveness of a treatment.

COMPLEMENTARY AND ALTERNATIVE MEDICINES

This volume has a large section dealing with complementary and alternative medicines (CAM) because they are widely used by people with any serious or chronic disease. Many studies have shown that three out of four MS patients use one or more alternative medicines and often seek help from alternative therapists, often while also using the conventional therapies prescribed by their physicians.

Dr. Marcia Angell and Dr. Jerome Kassirer, former editors of the *New England Journal of Medicine*, wrote that there cannot be two forms of medicine – conventional and alternative. "There is only medicine that has been adequately tested and medicine that has not, medicine that works and medicine that may or may not work." They argued that alternative medicines have been given a free ride, and when something is tested rigorously and shown to be safe and effective it does not matter whether it is alternative or conventional. Belief in alternative approaches may be strong, even when there are no studies to show effect or safety. They add, "But assertions, speculation, and testimonials do not substitute for evidence." The authors conclude, "Alternative treatments should be subjected to scientific testing no less rigorous that that required for conventional treatments."

ACQUIRING UP-TO-DATE INFORMATION ON MS

It is exciting to live in the "Information Age," but the methods available also bring confusion and even mis-information. This edition incorporates the new information, especially as it relates to the treatment and management of MS attacks, symptoms, and the underlying disease. As more people obtain information on the Internet, this book, which is sponsored by the MS International Federation, will also be available online (www.msif.org). This will also make it possible for the authors to rapidly update the text as important new information appears.

Other valuable sources of balanced, reliable, current information on MS include the national MS societies, which provide both printed information and Web sites.

Information on studies of conventional and alternative approaches to therapies are collected and evaluated by the Cochrane Controlled Trials Register, which lists thousands of randomized controlled trials and has conducted hundreds of meta-analyses on these trials. This information can be accessed through the Cochrane Library Web site (http://hiru.mcmaster.ca/COCH RANE.default.htm).

GENERAL HEALTH MEASURES
AND PREVENTATIVE APPROACHES

Although this book assesses various treatments that have been used in MS, it is important to recognize that drugs and procedures are only one aspect of the effective treatment and management of a person with MS. There are many ways that a person with MS can stay as healthy as possible, and cope and manage the many challenges that the disease brings, including:

1. Become informed about the disease, because through information you can best deal with questions, challenges, and issues as they arise.

2. Foster your support group of family, friends, and community.

3. Develop a good relationship with your physician and other health professionals.

4. Maintain normal activities and responsibilities as much as your symptoms and disease allow. Adopt a "rehabilitation approach" that emphasizes maintenance of activities despite the presence of symptoms and limitations. Good coping skills can be used to manage deficits and apply solutions to challenges.

5. Exercise.

6. Maintain a healthy diet.

7. Control weight.

8. Maintain a positive attitude that is wellness-oriented rather than disease-oriented.

9. Remember to pay attention to the basic health measures that are for everyone. Blood pressure measurement, breast examination, Pap tests, prostate examination, blood sugar level, cholesterol and lipids, and other

preventative approaches are equally important for a person who has MS.

10. MS affects the body, but the person living with MS has personal and spiritual resources that will allow them to remain strong and have a good quality of life.

Chapter 2

Treatment for an Acute Exacerbation

OVERVIEW

At least 80 to 85 percent of people with MS have an acute period of worsening (also called an *exacerbation, bout, attack,* or *relapse*) at some time. One of the most commonly used definitions of an exacerbation is the [sub] acute appearance of a neurologic abnormality that must be present for at least 24 hours in the absence of fever or infection. A wide variety of symptoms can occur during exacerbations. MRI scans taken at such times often show new active (gadolinium-enhancing) lesions in the brain or the reactivation or enlargement of old lesions.

Whereas quite some evidence points to the fact that exacerbations are the result of focal areas of inflammation in the CNS, little is known about what initiates exacerbations and which processes determine the level of recovery. Many studies have shown that there is an increased risk of exacerbations in the first 4 weeks after a systemic infection and that exacerbations following a systemic infection lead to more sustained damage than other exacerbations. There also seems to be a rather consistent association between stressful life events and subsequent exacerbations, but the identification of specific stressors so far has been unsuccessful. Another precipitating factor that has been identified is the early postpartum period.

A recent analysis of relapses that occurred in patients who were part of the placebo arm of clinical trials showed that 2 months after the initiation of a relapse about one-third of patients still had some measurable residual deficit.

Although most relapses remit spontaneously, many clinicians advise treatment for the relapses that have significant functional impact.

Corticosteroids have been the mainstay of treatment for the management of acute relapses for many years. They have immunomodulatory and antiinflammatory effects that restore the integrity of the blood–brain barrier, reduce edema, and possibly facilitate remyelination and improve axonal conduction. Corticosteroid therapy has been shown to shorten the duration and severity of the relapse and accelerate recovery, but there is no convincing evidence that the overall degree of recovery is improved or that the long-term course of the disease is altered.

Adrenocorticotropic hormone (ACTH, corticotropin) was the first agent demonstrated to be helpful in recovery from acute exacerbations. Brief courses of high-dose intravenous (IV) methylprednisolone (IVMP, 500–1000 mg/day for 3–5 days) have generally supplanted ACTH because of convenience, reliability, fewer side effects, and perhaps a more consistent and rapid onset of action.

Results of the Optic Neuritis Treatment Trial have been extrapolated by many neurologists to MS-associated relapses in general. In this study, 457 patients with acute optic neuritis were randomly assigned to receive 1000 mg of IVMP per day for 3 days followed by 1 mg of oral prednisone per kilogram per day for 11 days, 1 mg of oral prednisone per kilogram per day for 14 days, or oral placebo. The advantage of studying cases of optic neuritis is that very sensitive outcome measures (e.g., visual field, contrast sensitivity, color vision, and visual acuity) can be applied. The rate of recovery of vision was significantly faster in the IVMP-treated group, with the greatest benefits in patients with visual acuity of 20/40 or worse at entry. After 6 months there was no significant difference in visual acuity between the IVMP and placebo groups. Oral prednisone provided no benefit over placebo.

Unanticipated findings were that during the 6 to 24 months of follow-up, the risk of recurrent optic neuritis in either eye was increased with oral prednisone and that IVMP reduced by approximately 50 percent the risk of a new attack leading to the diagnosis of MS. This effect was most evident for patients at highest risk for subsequent relapse, that is, those with multiple brain lesions on MRI at entry into the study. These results should be interpreted with the understanding that this study was not designed to assess the effect of glucocorticoids on subsequent relapses and that the IVMP group was unblinded and lacked a placebo control. Differences between the treatment groups were no longer significant after 3 years, which suggests that IVMP at best delayed but did not stop the development of MS.

Magnetic resonance imaging follow-up studies have convincingly shown the effect of steroids, as evidenced by the reduction of gadolinium-enhancing lesions. However, this effect is only short-lived, and new enhancing lesions can develop within a week following treatment.

Despite the widespread use of corticosteroids as a treatment for relapses, very little is known about the optimal treatment regimen. The main controversies relate to the relative efficacy of the type of steroid (i.e., intramuscular ACTH versus IV steroids versus oral steroids), the optimal dosage for each route of administration, and whether a short course of IV treatment should be followed by a tapering regimen of orally administered corticosteroids.

Some clinicians substitute oral corticosteroid treatment for IVMP for the management of relapses mainly because of its easier route and reduced expense of administration. Data substantiating its equivalent benefit in acute relapse have been presented but are not very persuasive. Remarkably, in various studies—all being rather small—quite different dosage regimens of oral steroids have been applied.

Other antiinflammatory drugs, the so-called nonsteroidal antiinflammatory drugs (NSAIDs), including aspirin, indomethacin, ibuprofen, and naproxen, have not been shown to be of benefit in the treatment of MS relapses.

Conclusion: *A short course of IVMP remains the intervention of choice in patients with an acute exacerbation that warrants treatment. Prospective evidence indicates that it diminishes acute neurologic dysfunction; an effect on the long-term course of the disease has not been firmly established. It is unclear whether an oral taper of steroids would add any benefit.*

SPECIFIC AGENTS

Intravenous Methylprednisolone

As noted previously, it is common practice to employ a short course of corticosteroids to treat acute relapses of MS. Of the various approaches applied, the administration of IV methylprednisolone (IVMP) has become the most popular, especially because it can be given as a short course (typically 3–5 days), has a rapid onset of action, and is associated with relatively few side effects. Its use is now common practice in many clinics and hospitals on an outpatient basis. It should be given only under medical supervision because side effects, even though extremely rare, include psychosis, peptic ulceration, aseptic bone necrosis, infections, cardiac arrhythmias, and thrombo-embolism.

Some neurologists also employ periodic pulses of IVMP (e.g., once monthly) in patients with progressive MS, but there is no firm evidence that this has a favorable impact on the course of the disease, and there is an increased risk of side effects.

In the opinion of the Committee, a course of corticosteroids can be recommended for patients with exacerbations who have significant functional impact. Long-term use may be associated with significant serious side effects.

Intravenous Dexamethasone

Dexamethasone is another corticosteroid that shares many characteristics with methylprednisolone. Although the number of patients with MS exacerbations being treated with IV dexamethasone is substantially smaller than that being treated with IVMP, there is some evidence that its effects are comparable when given as a short course. In many countries its cost is substantially lower than that of IVMP.

> *In the opinion of the Committee, it is difficult to give a recommendation in the absence of carefully performed studies, but intravenous dexamethasone may represent a less expensive alternative to treatment with intravenous methylprednisolone.*

Intramuscular Adrenocorticotropic Hormone

Thirty-five years ago, short-term intramuscular (IM) adrenocorticotropic hormone ACTH given daily in high doses was shown to reduce the severity and shorten the duration of exacerbations. In more recent studies, claims have been made that IVMP works more quickly and effectively than ACTH, and most neurologists now prefer this treatment.

> *In the opinion of the Committee, intramuscular ACTH, although proven efficacious, is no longer the preferred treatment for MS exacerbations.*

Oral Steroids

There is conflicting evidence regarding the efficacy of oral steroids in the treatment of exacerbations. In the optic neuritis study referred to previously, there were more relapses in subsequent months in the oral prednisone group than in either the placebo-treated or the IVMP-treated group. Many people who have examined these data, however, reject the conclusion of the authors that oral prednisone was responsible for the increased later exacerbation rate.

A Danish study demonstrated the efficacy of oral methylprednisolone (MP) as a treatment for exacerbations. It compared the effects of oral MP therapy and placebo in patients with an episode lasting less than 4 weeks. Twenty-five patients received placebo, and 26 patients were given 500 mg oral MP once a day for 5 days, followed by a 10-day drug tapering period. Patients receiving MP did consistently better than those receiving placebo. At 8 weeks after the start of treatment, 32 percent of patients in the placebo group had improved by one Expanded Disability Status Scale (EDSS) point, whereas 65 percent of patients taking MP had a similar improvement.

Another study, performed in the United Kingdom, compared oral MP with IVMP: 80 patients with MS were treated within 4 weeks of the start of an exacerbation. Of these patients, 38 received IVMP (1000 mg/day for 3 days) and 42 received oral MP (48 mg/day for 7 days, followed by 24 mg/day for 7 days and 12 mg/day for the final 7 days). Hence, the cumulative dose of methylprednisolone was 3000 mg in the IV group and 588 mg in the oral group. The primary outcome was the difference between the two groups in improvement in the EDSS score of at least one full point after 4 weeks. No significant difference was found either with respect to this primary outcome or in any other measurement at any stage of the study. The main concerns regarding this study are that there was only a modest effect of treatment in both arms and that therefore a statistical type II error (real difference not being detected) is quite likely to occur. One must remember in this respect that statistical methods are tools that are predominantly developed to detect differences rather than to prove similarities: the absence of proof of difference is not equal to the proof of absence of difference.

It is extremely important that oral treatment with steroids not be prolonged because the complications of long-term treatment are well established. Complications include generalized puffiness, "moon face," psychosis, peptic ulceration, infections, and acne. Long-term use may even result in serious side effects, such as fractures related to bone softening, aseptic necrosis of bone, cataracts, hypertension, and adrenal insufficiency.

In the opinion of the Committee, treatment with oral steroids, even though it has recently gained some support, is not the preferred treatment for exacerbations, because only rather small studies (applying very different dosages) have been performed and it is not clear whether oral treatment, which in many regimens has to be prescribed longer than intravenous treatment, might increase the risk of side effects.

Intrathecal Steroids

In the opinion of the Committee, this therapy should not be used because of reported harmful effects.

Aspirin (Sodium Salicylate) and Nonsteroidal Antiinflammatory Drugs (Indomethacin, Phenylbutazone, Naproxen, Ibuprofen, and Fenoprofen)

These drugs are widely used to reduce inflammation, especially in arthritis. Proper evaluation of this type of drug in MS has not been done. A small study, however, suggests that ibuprofen is safe, although not effective in reducing the volume of active MS lesions seen on MRI. Ibuprofen and aspirin are being used to reduce early flu-like side effects of interferon beta and appear to be safe for the relief of discomfort.

In the opinion of the Committee, there appears to be no scientific basis for use of this therapy other than for the relief of early side effects associated with interferon therapy.

Plasmapheresis

During plasmapheresis (plasma exchange, or PE), blood is removed from the patient, and the liquid plasma and the cells are separated by centrifuge. The plasma (including many lymphocytes) is discarded and replaced by normal plasma or human albumin to avoid loss of protein and fluid. The "reconstituted" blood is then returned to the patient. This process may be repeated a number of times. It is believed that substances that can damage myelin and/or impair nerve conduction are removed in this way.

There remain numerous reports (most of them uncontrolled and reporting on only very small numbers of patients) that PE may be effective in fulminant acute syndromes of MS (or acute disseminated encephalomyelitis).

A randomized controlled trial was performed at the Mayo Clinic in the U.S.A. Thirty-six patients with recently acquired, severe neurological deficits resulting from attacks of inflammatory demyelinating disease, who failed to recover after treatment with IVMP, were treated with either plasma exchange or sham treatment. Moderate or greater improvement in neurological disability occurred during 8 of 19 courses of active treatment compared with 1 of 17 courses of sham treatment. Moderate or marked improvement was associated with the male sex, preserved reflexes, and early initiation of treatment. Successfully treated patients improved rapidly following treatment and the improvement was sustained.

In the opinion of the Committee, this therapy should be considered for those rare cases that present with acute, fulminant symptomatology and do not respond to intravenous steroids.

Intravenous Immunoglobulin

Intravenous immunoglobulin (IVIG) is pooled human IgG that is presumed to alter the immune system by various mechanisms (also see page 41). A small, randomized trial testing the efficacy of adding IVIG to IVMP in the treatment of relapses was performed in the Netherlands. A beneficial effect of IVIG could not be demonstrated.

In the opinion of the Committee, IVIG should not be added to IVMP in patients with an acute exacerbation.

Guide to Further Reading

- Barnes D, Hughes RAC, Morris RW, et al. Randomized trial of oral and intravenous methylprednisolone in acute relapses of multiple sclerosis. *Lancet* 1997; 349:902–906.

- Beck RW, Cleary PA, Anderson MM, et al. A randomized, controlled trial of corticosteroids in the treatment of acute optic neuritis. The Optic Neuritis Study Group. *N Engl J Med* 1992; 326:581–588.

- Beck RW, Cleary PA, Trobe JD, et al. The effect of corticosteroids for acute optic neuritis on the subsequent development of multiple sclerosis. The Optic Neuritis Study Group. *N Engl J Med* 1993; 329:1764–1769.

- Buljevac D, Flach HZ, Hop WCJ, et al. Prospective study on the relationship between infections and multiple sclerosis exacerbations. *Brain* 2002; 125:952–960.

- Confavreux C, Hutchinson M, Hours MM, et al. Rate of pregnancy-related relapse in multiple sclerosis. *N Engl J Med* 1998; 339:285–291.

- Keegan M, Pineda AA, McClelland RL, et al. Plasma exchange for severe attacks of CNS demyelination: predictors of response. *Neurology* 2002; 58:143–146.

- Lublin FD, Baier M, Cutter G. Effect of relapses on development of residual deficit in multiple sclerosis. *Neurology* 2003; 61:1528–32.

- Milligan NG, Newcombe R, Compston DAS. A double-blind controlled trial of high dose methylprednisolone in patients with multiple sclerosis. 1. Clinical effects. *J Neurol Neurosurg Psychiatry* 1986; 50:511–516.

- Mohr DC, Hart SL, Julian L, et al. Association between stressful life events and exacerbation in multiple sclerosis: a meta-analysis. *BMJ* 2004; 328:731–735.

- Sellebjerg F, Frederiksen JL, Nielsen PM, Olesen J. Double-blind, randomized, placebo-controlled study of oral, high-dose methylprednisolone in attacks of MS. *Neurology* 1998; 51:529–534.

- Thompson AJ, Kennard C, Swash M, et al. Relative efficacy of intravenous methylprednisolone and ACTH in the treatment of acute relapse in MS. *Neurology* 1989; 39:969–971.

- Visser LH, Beekman R, Tijssen CC, et al. A randomized, double-blind, placebo-controlled pilot study of IV immune globulins in combination with IV methylprednisolone in the treatment of relapses in patients with MS. *Multiple Sclerosis* 2004; 10:89–91.

- Weinshenker BG, O'Brien PC, Petterson TM, et al. A randomized trial of plasma exchange in acute central nervous system inflammatory demyelinating disease. *Ann Neurol* 1999; 46:878–886.

Chapter 3

Treatments That Affect the Long-Term Course of the Disease ("Disease-Modifying Therapy")

The goal of therapy in patients with MS is to prevent relapses and progressive worsening of the disease. The documentation of therapeutic advances in MS is dependent on large, randomized, controlled clinical trials because of the highly variable and unpredictable course of the disease and the difficulty in precisely measuring neurologic disability.

Immunosuppressive drugs that dampen certain aspects of immune system function were used initially, but they have never found widespread acceptance because the various studies have met with limited success as a result of variable efficacy and considerable toxicity (especially with long-term use), mainly because of the induction of bone marrow suppression.

More recently, large, randomized, controlled trials have been performed with substances that should be seen as immune *modulators* rather than as immune *suppressors*. These studies have led to the regulatory approval of a series of "disease-modifying" agents [Avonex®, Betaseron® (Betaferon® in Europe), Copaxone®, and Rebif® worldwide, and mitoxantrone (Novantrone®) and Tysabri® in North America]. Although there is some evidence for a reduction in the rate of progression of neurologic impairment and disability, none of these agents have been shown to achieve a sustained remission, complete halt of further progression, or substantially alleviate long-standing disability.

Therefore, in individual patients, decisions to initiate treatment should be based on the course of that patient's disease. Patients (and often family members) should actively participate in every treatment decision. There is considerable inter-individual variability between patients. Faced with the same clinical scenario and the same, careful review of what is known about the value of the approved medications, some patients will decide to delay treatment, whereas others will choose to be started on treatment as soon as the diagnosis has been established. On the one hand, approximately 10 to 20 percent of patients have relatively benign disease, so not every patient may require disease-modifying therapy. On the other hand, treatment should not be postponed until after persistent neurologic deficits have occurred because none of the available compounds reverse fixed deficits. Disease-modifying therapy should be considered early in the course for patients with an unfavorable prognosis, but, unfortunately, the rate and pattern of progression of disease cannot be reliably predicted at initial assessment. Although long-term follow-up of monosymptomatic patients indicates that the likelihood of a second clinical event and the development of disability increases with certain clinical characteristics (progressive course of disease, sphincter or motor symptoms at onset, male sex, or high attack frequency within the first years) as well as with the lesion load on brain MRI, determining the exact future prospectives for a given individual is still not possible because the prognostic value of these factors is only modest.

Before long-term therapies are implemented, it is extremely important that counseling about realistic objectives regarding efficacy and side effects takes place, because overly optimistic expectations may complicate treatment. Patients who understand these issues are more likely to remain compliant with the medications once the decision has been reached to commence treatment.

FROM BETTER UNDERSTANDING
TO BETTER TREATMENT

Although the cause of MS is not known, it is generally believed that environmental factors (possibly viral infections) trigger an immunologically mediated process in individuals of a certain genetic background. Genetic factors involved in disease susceptibility probably consist of multiple interacting genes.

Because current theories favor the idea that MS is an immunologic disease, a brief review of the immune system is important. The normal function of the immune system is to recognize and repel foreign invaders, such as bacteria, viruses, and other foreign substances (antigens). Normally, the immune system recognizes "self" components and does not destroy them by mistake. An "autoimmune" disease occurs when this system fails to recognize a "self" component as such and attacks it. In the case of MS, strong evidence points to a mistaken attack on the myelin that surrounds most neurons.

Almost 60 years ago it was shown that injections of brain extracts in animals would make some of them develop an inflammatory disease of the central nervous system called *experimental allergic encephalomyelitis* (EAE). This disease was quite similar to one that was accidentally produced in some humans with an old preparation of rabies vaccine containing fragments of myelin. Post-rabies vaccine encephalomyelitis, in turn, was quite similar pathologically to occasional forms of postinfectious encephalomyelitis appearing in a few unlucky children after naturally occurring measles, rubella, chickenpox, and occasionally other viruses.

Postinfectious encephalomyelitis in humans is not a recurrent disease; it occurs only once. Later it was shown that a chronic relapsing form of EAE could be produced in some genetically susceptible animals. These animals recovered from attacks of paralysis only to develop symptoms weeks or months later in a manner similar to development of MS symptoms. Moreover, pathologic changes in the CNS of such animals are quite similar to those seen in MS.

However, there are important differences between MS and chronic EAE. The antigen is clearly myelin or a myelin component in EAE; the antigen in MS is still unknown. Another important difference is that EAE is easily inhibited and suppressed by a number of drugs that seem to have little impact on MS. A recent observation that the presence of antibodies to myelin antigens at the time of the initial clinical presentation (e.g., in the setting of a "clinically isolated syndrome") increases the chances of an early conversion to clinically definite MS needs to be validated.

The immune system is complex. Its basic units are two kinds of white blood cells located in the thymus, spleen, and lymph nodes. These cells circulate to all parts of the body by way of the blood and the lymph. The larger cells are *macrophages* (Greek: "big-eaters"). They function by engulfing and disposing of debris. They also secrete chemicals known as *proteases*, which are capable of destroying myelin, prostaglandins, and free oxygen radicals, which, in turn, have profound effects on inflammation and immune function. The smaller cells are *lymphocytes* and they come in several varieties. *B lymphocytes* are processed in the bone marrow and become antibody-producing cells. The more numerous *T lymphocytes* are processed mostly in the thymus gland. They become activated when exposed to an antigen to which they are reactive; the cell becomes metabolically more active, enlarges, and secretes a group of chemicals called *cytokines*. Some of the functions of cytokines are to promote enlargement of lymphocyte populations, activate macrophages, increase blood flow and edema of tissue, and attract other types of white blood cells to the area. Interferon gamma is one such cytokine secreted by activated T cells. This substance facilitates antigen recognition, and its use in the treatment of MS has been associated with an increase in the frequency of exacerbations.

Current evidence suggests that cytokines can basically be divided into *pro-inflammatory* cytokines, such as tumor necrosis factor (TNF-alpha), and interferon gamma (IFN-gamma), which may be directly responsible for tissue damage in MS, and *anti-*

inflammatory cytokines, such as interleukin-4 (IL-4), interleukin-10 (IL-10), and transforming growth factor beta (TGF-beta), which suppress or inhibit disease.

Many B lymphocytes also exist in and around the MS plaques, but they are relatively uncommon in the cerebrospinal fluid (CSF). They are the source of local immunoglobulin production. Immunoglobulins are antibodies, but in the case of MS the target antigen is unknown, and efforts to find the antigen by studying the antibodies have been largely unsuccessful so far.

It has been clearly established from neuropathologic studies of MS lesions that it is against this background of inflammatory cells and cytokines that active demyelination takes place. Traditionally, inflammation and demyelination are considered to be the hallmark of MS lesions (MS is often listed as an "inflammatory demyelinating disease"). Recent studies, however, have reemphasized the importance of damage to the neural cells themselves ("axonal damage") as a major correlate of permanent clinical deficits.

Therapeutic approaches aim at utilizing the increased level of understanding of the immune system; for example, by administering antiinflammatory cytokines to patients with MS or by developing strategies that inhibit proinflammatory cytokines. However, the complex network of the immune system with mutually interdependent factors and mechanisms, which can vary between different phases of the disease, limits the ability to predict the effect of an immune intervention once it is given to a patient. Additional complexity is introduced by the emerging pathologic heterogeneity of MS that apparently encompasses a spectrum from highly destructive cellular lesions and demyelinative processes with or without significant cellular involvement, to primary oligodendrogliopathies.

Given our limited understanding of disease pathogenesis in general, and in a given person with the disease, concrete therapeutic advances in MS are critically dependent on clinical trials. Because of the highly variable and unpredictable course of the disease and the difficulty in precisely measuring neurologic disability, these trials traditionally require large numbers of patients and long periods of follow-up.

DRUGS APPROVED FOR USE IN MS

Interferon Beta (Avonex®, Betaseron®/Betaferon®, and Rebif®)

Interferons (IFNs) are small molecules (cytokines) produced by cells of the immune system in response to a variety of inducers, especially viruses. They have been demonstrated to have antiviral, antiproliferative, and immunomodulating properties and are divided into two types: type 1 includes alpha and beta IFN; type 2 is gamma IFN. Interferons were initially considered for the treatment of MS because of a presumed viral pathogenesis. There was some evidence for a decrease in the level of IFN gamma in the CSF of MS patients, and a pilot study was performed to assess the safety and efficacy of IFNs. This trial was prematurely terminated because of an unexpected increase in the relapse rate. The negative result of this trial provided an important clue to the understanding of the pathogenesis of MS, and subsequent studies focused on the effects of type 1 IFNs because they were found to have a number of immunomodulatory effects that were quite the opposite of those of IFN gamma. IFN alpha and beta use the same receptor and have similar effects and a high degree of homology.

Initially, a number of studies reported limited efficacy for intrathecally, subcutaneously, and intramuscularly administered type 1 IFN in decreasing the frequency of exacerbations in relapsing-remitting MS (RRMS). In several of these studies, these effects were shown to be reversible, with the return of markers of disease activity to baseline after discontinuation of treatment. This supported the hypothesis that the observed changes were indeed the result of IFN therapy. Therefore, further studies were performed, which took advantage of the availability of recombinant IFN and abandoned natural IFN. At present, two forms of recombinant IFN beta (1a [Avonex® and Rebif®] and 1b [Betaseron®/Betaferon®]) have been approved by regulatory authorities. Each are made by recombinant DNA technology in tissue culture and are highly purified before use. IFN beta-1a is a glycosylated, recombinant mammalian-cell product, with an amino acid sequence identical to that of natural interferon beta. IFN beta-1b is a nonglycosylated recombinant bacterial-cell product in which serine is substituted for cysteine at position 17.

Interferon Beta-1a

Two forms of IFN beta-1a were subject to investigation in large clinical trials: Avonex® and Rebif®. Avonex® was initially tested in a trial involving 301 patients with relapsing MS and mild to moderate neurologic impairment (baseline disability score on the EDSS 1.0–3.5). Treatment consisted of weekly intramuscular (IM) injections (6 million units, or 30 mcg) or placebo for up to 2 years, the dose and timing of administration being based on the serum level of $beta_2$-microglobulin and the occurrence of side effects. The principal outcome measure was the length of time to progression of disability, defined as a worsening from baseline of at least one point on the EDSS that persisted for at least 6 months.

The study was terminated when it was recognized that the drop-out rate was less than anticipated. At the time the trial was stopped, 57 percent of enrolled patients had completed 2 years, and 77 percent had been followed up for 18 months. Despite this early termination, the IFN beta-1a–treated patients were significantly less likely to reach the primary outcome, the probability being about 21 percent in the treatment group, and 33 percent in the placebo group for those who completed 2 years of therapy. An 18 percent reduction in exacerbations was noted for the treated group, and those patients who completed 2 years had one-third fewer exacerbations. The treatment effect was supported by a reduction of gadolinium enhancement and new or enlarging lesions on annual MRIs. A significant difference between the treatment groups, however, was not found for the total brain lesion load.

The clinical significance of the beneficial effect of IFN beta-1a on disease progression at the lower EDSS scores has been endorsed by the findings of a post hoc statistical analysis of the disability outcomes data obtained in this study. Sensitivity calculations indicated that the primary outcome parameter was robust to changes in definitions of EDSS progression and that the proportion of patients progressing to EDSS milestones of 4.0 and 6.0 was significantly lower in the IFN-treated patients. This study was pivotal in the decision of the FDA to license this agent for clinical use.

In a recent placebo-controlled study involving 383 individuals with a first episode suggestive for MS and specific MRI features that are prognostically unfavorable, Avonex® significantly prolonged the time to a second episode. Early use of IFN reduced MRI indicators of subclinical disease activity, but the trial was too short to provide insights about any possible benefits in delaying or reducing disability. Subsequent analyses showed that half of the treated patients continued to show MRI evidence of probable disease activity during the first 18 months of treatment, suggesting that even early treatment did not completely suppress the illness. This study was influential in North American and European regulatory authorities approving this agent for use in this subset of patients at risk of MS.

A large study investigating the effects of Avonex® on disease progression in patients with secondary progressive MS ("IMPACT") failed to demonstrate a favorable effect on disability progression as measured by the EDSS, but did suggest possible slowing of worsening using an allegedly more sensitive outcome measure (the MS Functional Composite Measure). An additional phase-three study in RRMS suggested that 30 and 60 mg doses of IFN β-1a (once weekly IM) are comparable.

Rebif® was investigated in a number of studies, including one in which 560 patients with active relapsing-remitting disease and mild to moderate disability (EDSS 0–5) were randomized to treatment with IFN beta-1a 6 MIU (22 mcg), 12 MIU (44 mcg), or placebo, given subcutaneously three times a week (tiw) for 2 years. The primary end point for this study was the relapse rate. At the end of the study, 95 percent of the patient data was available for analysis. The results showed that, compared with placebo, IFN beta-1a significantly decreased the number (by 27 percent and 33 percent, with 22 mcg and 44 mcg, respectively) and severity of exacerbations, and increased the time to the first and second relapses. It also increased the percentage of patients who were relapse-free during the study.

In addition, IFN beta-1a prolonged the time to confirmed progression as measured with EDSS scores (1.0 point confirmed at 3 months). Furthermore, there was a significant reduction in the disease activity on MRI (gadolinium-enhancing lesions, new lesions, or enlarging T2 lesions) as well as on total T2 lesion load in patients receiving active treatment compared with those given placebo. The placebo group showed an accumulation of approximately 11 percent in lesion load over the 2 years, whereas there was a decrease of about 1 percent among patients receiving 6 MIU and a decrease of almost 4 percent in the 12 MIU group.

After 2 years, patients initially receiving placebo were randomized to blinded IFN beta-1a 22 mcg or 44 mcg three tiw, whereas all other patients continued blinded treatment with their originally assigned dose of IFN beta-1a. Clinical and MRI benefit continued for both doses up to 4 years, with 44 mcg tiw being superior to 22 mcg tiw for some of the outcome measures applied. Outcomes also were consistently better for patients who were treated for 4 years than for patients in the crossover groups, who only received active treatment during years 3 and 4.

Another study with Rebif® compared three different doses of IFN beta-1a administered once weekly with placebo, showing increasing treatment effect with increasing dose.

A large placebo-controlled trial in secondary progressive MS (SPMS) reported that Rebif® given three times weekly failed to have a significant effect on disease progression, as defined by the time to confirmed neurologic deterioration (1-point increase) on the EDSS present for at least 3 months. This study demonstrated, however, that this drug reduced both clinical relapses and MRI evidence of worsening, suggesting continued biological activity in this patient cohort. The lack of benefit on clinical disability, however, suggests that the benefit of Rebif® in this patient group is low. A low dose (22 mcg sc once weekly) reduced the likelihood of a second episode in the subsequent 2 years in patients with a first episode suggestive of MS who have prognostically unfavorable MRI features. This finding was similar to that reported earlier for weekly IM IFN β-1a (Avonex®) despite the very low dose of the drug.

One recent study ("Evidence") reported that three times weekly 44 mcg sc IFN β-1a (Rebif®) more effectively reduced relapse rate, compared with once weekly IM (Avonex®) administration, although it was associated with a greater frequency of neutralizing antibody formation (see below). This study was too brief to provide disability information.

Interferon Beta-1b

Interferon beta-1b was initially tested in a multicenter U.S. trial involving 372 patients with RRMS and mild to moderate disability (EDSS up to 5.5). Treatment consisted of either 8 MIU (250 mcg) or 1.6 MIU (50 mcg) of IFN beta-1b or placebo given by subcutaneous injection every other day. The primary outcome was the relapse rate. Compared with placebo, treatment with the higher dose reduced the relapse rate by 31 percent, increased the time to first relapse and the proportion of patients who were relapse-free, and reduced by about 50 percent the number of patients who had moderate and severe relapses. There was, however, no difference in changes in EDSS scores between treatment groups. The patients in the placebo group had a mean increase of 17 percent in the total lesion load on brain MRI at 3 years compared with a mean decrease of 6 percent in those receiving high-dose IFN beta-1b. In addition, there was a significant reduction in disease activity as measured by the analysis of new or enlarging lesions on serial MRIs.

A second multicenter trial of IFN beta-1b was performed in Europe, including 718 patients with SPMS (EDSS at inclusion 3.0–6.5) whose disease had been clinically active in the 2 years preceding the study (defined as either two relapses or deterioration of at least 1 EDSS point). Treatment consisted of either 8 MIU of IFN beta-1b or placebo subcutaneously on alternate days over 3 years. The primary outcome was the time to confirmed neurologic deterioration, defined as a 1-point increase on the EDSS present for at least 3 months. In this study, for EDSS scores of 6.0 and higher, a change of 0.5 point was considered to be equal to 1.0 point for scores lower than 6.0. A prospectively planned interim analysis for efficacy was performed after all patients had completed at least 24 months of treatment. An alpha level of 0.0133 was predetermined for the intent-to-treat analysis of the primary end point.

Based on this interim analysis, the independent Advisory Board recommended that the study be stopped because there was a highly significant difference regarding the primary end point ($p \leq 0.0008$). The delay in progression was within a range of 9 to 12 months. This effect was seen in patients both with and without superimposed relapses before or during the study, and it was consistent across all baseline EDSS levels studied. Significant reductions in time to require wheelchair use (EDSS 7.0), number of steroid courses given, and number of MS-related hospitalizations were also observed. Effects on relapse rate and MRI were consistent with the findings in the relapsing-remitting population. Whereas the mean lesion volume increased by about 8 percent at 2 years, the mean lesion load in the active treatment group decreased by about 5 percent. In a subcohort of 125 patients a marked and significant reduction of new and enhancing lesions could be demonstrated for two 6-month periods of frequent scanning (months 1–6 and 19–24). Additional MRI measures suggested, however, that this agent does not prevent the progression of cerebral atrophy. This study was the first to report a significant impact of any disease modifying treatment on the accumulation of disability in SPMS.

Strikingly, this favorable effect on disability progression could not be confirmed in a North American study of IFN beta-1b in SPMS. Even though this study tested the same therapeutic agent and dose, and both studies had similar (although not identical) entry criteria and study designs, no treatment benefit was seen on the time to confirmed progression of disability.

Effects on relapse- and MRI-related outcomes were consistently in favor of interferon beta-1b treated patients, a result consistent with earlier clinical trials.

A large, but unblinded, study ("Incomin") compared IFN beta-1b, 8 MIU on alternate days with once weekly IM (Avonex®) in patients with RRMS. In the same way as the "Evidence" study (see above), it concluded that relapses and MRI evidence of disease activity were less likely with more frequent dosing of IFN beta.

Side Effects Associated with Interferon Beta Treatment

Treatment with IFN beta usually is well tolerated. Side effects depend partially on the dosage used and the route of administration. For all preparations mentioned, patients can experience flu-like reactions such as fever, myalgia, chills, and general discomfort for 24 to 48 hours after each injection, especially during the first months of treatment. These symptoms, however, generally are mild to moderate in severity and tend to decrease over time. Symptom management requires simple practical techniques such as dose escalation (some experts advocate giving a low dose of prednisone during the early weeks of initiating this agent), bedtime dosing, and the use of acetaminophen (paracetamol in Europe) or ibuprofen. The frequency of injection-site reactions (redness, tenderness, and swelling) is also initially high, almost exclusively in those patients who receive treatment by subcutaneous injection. Reactions can be managed by improving injection technique (e.g., warming the solution to room temperature, icing the injection site after each injection, and avoiding intradermal injections and excessive sun exposure) and maintaining site rotation. Injection-site necrosis occurs in about 5 percent of patients. In earlier studies, there was a suggestion that treatment with IFN beta could lead to depression or suicide attempts, but this was not supported by subsequent studies. Some people with MS report an initial worsening of symptoms during the first weeks of IFN therapy; an increase in spasticity has been reported in patients with primary and secondary progressive disease. IFN beta can also cause elevations in liver function tests, lymphopenia, or anemia. Some reports address the potential for severe autoimmune disease (thyroiditis, Grave's disease, and hypothyroidism) after administration of IFN beta. Blood count and liver function are generally measured at baseline, then monthly for 3 months, and then every 3 months thereafter. The dose or frequency of administration in patients with elevated liver enzymes or neutropenia (rarely anemia) is reduced, but treatment is usually not discontinued. There are isolated reports that IFN beta administration may be followed by myasthenia gravis, rheumatoid arthritis, systemic lupus erythematous, inflammatory arthritis, urticaria, Raynaud's phenomenon, worsening of psoriasis, anaphylaxis, and intracerebral hemorrhage, but the association with IFN treatment often is unclear. Overall, the percentage of patients discontinuing treatment because of serious or intolerable side effects is low.

Unresolved Issues Related to Treatment with Interferon Beta

Although a number of studies have provided supportive evidence that IFN beta favorably influences the short-term course of MS, the long-term effects on the development of disability are not known. Also, there have been no conclusive studies in PPMS, and the preliminary data suggests that the (small) potential impact is outweighed by side-effects.

Another important consideration is the propensity for IFN beta to stimulate the formation of neutralizing antibodies (NABs), which might depend on a number of variables, including a dose-administered (greater risk with the lower dose of sc IFN β-1a) route of administration (lower risk for IM versus sc route), frequency of administration (lower risk with once weekly administration), and type of IFN beta used. A number of studies suggest that the rate of NAB formation seems to be less in the IFN beta-1a trials (5–20 percent as compared with 25 to 35 percent for IFN beta-1b), but the fact that different assays were used in some of these studies must be taken into account. There are reports that the development of NABs is associated with reduced effectiveness (relapse rate reduction). This remains a great concern, but it seems that with time antibody levels may disappear in many patients. Because of the uncertain validity of the assay of NABs and the limited study of their consequences, everyday clinical practice decisions based on the presence or absence of NABs cannot yet be made with confidence.

The cost of therapy, currently at least the equivalent of U.S. $10,000, requires a careful cost-benefit analysis. It is still not known when treatment ideally should be initiated or whether it should be discontinued at some point. For individual patients, these costs and the still rather limited information on long-term risks may outweigh the benefits, especially if they have benign disease. Present guidelines for stopping therapy are related to side effects, a desire to become pregnant, and perceived inefficacy as documented by relapses or progression of disability. A recent report suggests that both clinical relapses during treatment with IFN beta and new MRI lesion activity correlate with poor response to treatment.

Clarifying the mechanism of action also is of great importance, not only because it could guide further research with respect to other treatment modalities that could be used (alone or in combination with IFN beta), but also because it might allow discrimination between those patients who are likely to respond to the drug and those who are not. Interferons inhibit T-lymphocyte and monocyte activation and proliferation, reduce IFN gamma and MHC-II expression, increase IL-10 production, down-regulate antigen presentation, reduce lymphocyte migration and blood–brain barrier permeability, and alter the body's response to viral infections.

> *In the opinion of the Committee, treatment with interferon beta should be recommended for patients with active relapsing disease. At this time it is not possible to decide which, if any, of the interferon beta preparations should be preferred. There is some indication that more frequent and higher-dosed interferon beta has superior efficacy, but for some patients once weekly intramuscular administration seems to be better tolerated. For patients in the (secondary) progressive phase of the disease, the recommendation to initiate treatment is much weaker. The relatively negative results of three of the four pivotal trials in secondary progressive MS suggest that this class of treatment likely has little meaningful effect in slowing clinical disability in this cohort of patients.*

Glatiramer Acetate (Copaxone®)

Glatiramer acetate (previously called *copolymer-1*) is a synthetic copolymer composed of alanine, glutamine, lysine, and tyrosine, with some immunologic similarities to one of the important myelin components, myelin basic protein (MBP), without itself being encephalitogenic. The observation that it inhibits the animal model EAE prompted double-blind clinical trials.

The largest of these trials was a 2-year, double-blind trial carried out in the United States involving 251 patients with RRMS (baseline EDSS 0–5). Treatment consisted of daily subcutaneous injections of 20 mg of glatiramer acetate or placebo. The primary end point was the annualized relapse rate, which was reduced by 29 percent in the group receiving active treatment. There also was a reduction in the percentage of patients remaining relapse-free and the median time to first relapse. A statistically significant favorable effect on EDSS progression was evident only with a less conservative data analysis, thereby providing a trend, but not significant proof for an effect on progression of disability. There has been a lack of MRI data for some years, but recently data from a 9-month, double-blind, placebo-controlled trial with a primary MRI end point demonstrated that glatiramer acetate administration is followed by a delayed reduction of blood–brain barrier permeability (peak effect is after a number of months rather than a few weeks for the interferons) and a suppression of new lesion development. This finding may result from the effect of glatiramer acetate in down-regulating the immune response rather than a specific effect on the blood-brain barrier. Glatiramer acetate does not reduce T cell migration.

Long-term follow-up of the patients who participated in this trial suggests that glatiramer might have a favorable impact on long-term disability progression, but the interpretation of these follow-up data is significantly limited by patients being lost to follow-up. A large trial (Promise Trial) to evaluate the effects of glatiramer acetate over 3 years in patients with PPMS was terminated at a preplanned interim analysis because a treatment effect was very unlikely to occur during the remainder of the study.

Adverse effects of glatiramer acetate are usually mild, and include localized injection-site reactions and a systemic reaction occurring within minutes of administration of the drug (associated with chest pain, palpitations, or dyspnea, and always resolving spontaneously in less than 30 minutes). This reaction occurs in a small minority of patients, usually only once, and not necessarily after the first injection. Occasional patients develop lipoatrophy at injection sites and lymphadenopathy has been reported. Glatiramer acetate does not induce changes in liver function, blood count, or thyroid function. Consequently, the regular monitoring of blood work that is necessary with the IFNS is not needed for patients treated with glatiramer acetate.

Serum antibodies to glatiramer acetate also develop, but their presence seems to have no effect on the clinical benefit.

The apparent effect on reducing relapse rate might be due to blocking of the presentation of certain myelin antigens to T lymphocytes. Other proposed mechanisms of action include the induction of suppressor cells that migrate systemically to modulate the immune response within the nervous system ("bystander suppression"). Of great interest are the observations that glatiramer acetate-reactive cells may secrete growth factors that may enhance repair within the MS plaque, and that anti-glatiramer acetate antibodies may enhance remyelination.

In the opinion of the Committee, glatiramer acetate constitutes an effective therapy for patients with relapsing-remitting MS. Recent suggestions that the drug slows the rate of disability progression need to be confirmed by additional studies. Some patients seem to tolerate glatiramer acetate better than interferon beta during the first months of treatment.

Mitoxantrone

Mitoxantrone is an antineoplastic agent that exerts potent immunomodulatory effects, including suppression of B cell immunity and reduction of T cell numbers. Mitoxantrone shows considerably less acute toxicity than many other anticancer drugs, the most serious side effects being irreversible cardiotoxicity (cardiomyopathy) and lymphoma. Recently three studies were published in which the effects of this compound were investigated in MS.

A French multicenter study of 42 patients with very active disease compared treatment with either mitoxantrone (20 mg IV monthly) and methylprednisolone (1 g IV monthly), or methylprednisolone alone for 6 months. Blinded analysis of MRI data showed a significant and very strong suppression of disease activity in favor of the mitoxantrone-treated patients; unblinded clinical assessments also favored the mitoxantrone group.

An Italian study enrolled 51 patients with relapsing-remitting disease in a randomized, placebo-controlled design (8 mg/

m2 IV monthly for 1 year) of 2 years duration. A trend toward reduction in disease activity as measured with clinical and MRI parameters was also found.

More recently, the results of a European multicenter, placebo-controlled, randomized, blinded, phase III study were presented. Patients with SPMS ($n = 194$) were randomized to either of two doses of mitoxantrone (5 mg/m^2 or 12 mg/m^2) or placebo, given intravenously every 3 months for 2 years. A significant beneficial effect on relapse rate and disability progression was found in the absence of severe toxicity. MRI data confirmed the beneficial effect on disease activity, although the full analysis of the MRI data has not yet been published. Treatment was well tolerated. This report convinced the FDA to license mitoxantrone for secondary (chronic) progressive, progressive relapsing, or worsening relapsing-remitting MS.

Mitoxantrone causes mild nausea (usually without vomiting), mild alopecia, amenorrhea in up to 25 percent of premenopausal women, and dose-related bone marrow suppression. When considering treatment with mitoxantrone, it is extremely important that patients with (risk factors for) cardiac disease be excluded and that (depending on the dosage regimen used) blood counts and urine samples be taken. Echocardiographic studies should also be performed every 6 months. No patient should receive an accumulative dose exceeding 100–120 mg/m^2, and the drug should be discontinued if there are symptoms or clinical (or echo) findings of reduced cardiac contractility. There are a number of recent reports that mitoxantrone may induce leukemia, presumably through its profound immunosuppressive activity.

In the opinion of the Committee, available evidence studies suggest that mitoxantrone is effective in reducing disease activity in MS. It should be considered a second-line drug to be used in patients with aggressive MS (frequent relapses with incomplete recovery) who have failed to respond adequately to the interferons or glatiramer acetate. The issue of long-term safety is likely to limit the duration of treatment.

Natalizumab (Tysabri®)

Natalizumab (Tysabri®) is a humanized monoclonal antibody against the α4 chain of α4β1 integrin. Monoclonal antibodies are antibodies that can be very specifically targeted to certain molecules; they thereby represent a way of inducing selective immunomodulation. "Humanized" means that a murine antibody clone has been grafted to a human framework in order to reduce its immunogenicity.

Integrins are a family of molecules that are part of the adhesion molecules, which are essential in virtually all cellular interactions of immune cells. The glycoprotein α4β1 integrin, also known as *very late antigen 4*, or *VLA-4*, is expressed on the surface of activated white blood cells and is an important mediator of cell adhesion and transendothelial migration. It plays a crucial role in determining whether inflammatory cells can enter the brain. Observations in animals with EAE have shown that preventing inflammatory cells from entering the brain can be an effective way to prevent new inflammatory demyelinating lesion formation.

In a randomized, double-blind phase II trial, 213 patients with relapsing MS were treated with 3 mg of IV natalizumab per kilogram of body weight, 6 mg per kilogram, or placebo every 28 days for 6 months. Treatment significantly reduced the number of new brain lesions on monthly gadolinium enhanced MRI during the 6-month treatment period, the primary endpoint of the study, as well as significantly reduced the number of clinical relapses. Treated patients were less likely to develop MRI evidence of T1 "black holes," perhaps indicating an important reduction in irreversible tissue injury. The treatment benefit disappeared shortly after the treatment was stopped. During the 6-month follow-up period, there was no significant difference in the number of active scans and reported relapses between the placebo and treated arms.

Very recently, the results of two large phase III trials with natalizumab were presented. The AFFIRM study is a placebo-controlled study involving 942 participants worldwide. Participants were randomly assigned to receive either a 300 mg IV infusion of natalizumab or placebo every 4 weeks. After 1 year, those on active therapy showed a statistically significant, 66 percent reduction in relapse rate. In the SENTINEL study, natalizumab was compared to placebo in patients who used interferon beta-1a (Avonex®). The 1,171 participants worldwide who continued to experience disease activity during treatment with interferon beta-1a were randomly assigned to add natalizumab or placebo. After 1 year, the participants who were treated with both natalizumab and interferon beta-1a experienced a 54 percent reduction in the rate of clinical relapses compared to those on placebo and interferon beta-1a. MRI outcomes (new active lesions and gadolinium-enhancement) also were consistently in favor of natalizumab-treated patients in both studies. During 12 months of therapy, the treatment was well-tolerated and safe. Serious infections such as pneumonia and urinary tract infections were slightly more frequent in natalizumab-treated patients. Natalizumab has been associated with hypersensitivity reactions, including serious systemic reactions, which occurred at an incidence of less than 1 percent of patients. The long-term safety of natalizumab is unknown.

The FDA has approved natalizumab to reduce the frequency of relapses in the relapsing forms of MS because it appears to provide substantial benefit, even though the complete set of results from AFFIRM and SENTINEL, both being 2-year studies, is not yet available.

In the opinion of the Committee, natalizumab seems to be an important additional treatment option. The drug is very effective and well-tolerated, but long-term safety is unknown. A full assessment of the drug can only be made after scientific publication of the study data, including the 2-year results.

While this publication is in press, all administration of natalizumab has been suspended worldwide due to the occur-

rence of three cases of progressive multifocal leucoencephalopathy, a cerebral infection with the JC-virus that is often lethal.

TREATMENTS THAT ARE NOT SPECIFICALLY APPROVED FOR MS BUT ARE BEING USED IN CERTAIN PARTS OF THE WORLD

A number of other treatment modalities, most of which are accepted treatments for inflammatory, immune-mediated diseases outside the CNS, have also been investigated in MS. Although they have not yet been licensed for use in MS, evidence in favor of or against their use is reviewed in this section.

Intravenous Immunoglobulin

Intravenous immunoglobulin (IVIG) is pooled human IgG that is presumed to alter the immune system by various mechanisms.

Whereas some smaller studies initially failed to reveal clear evidence of efficacy, an Austrian multicenter study provided evidence that monthly-administered, low-dose IVIG is effective and well tolerated. A group of 148 patients with relapsing-remitting disease (EDSS 1–6) were randomized to receive monthly doses of IVIG (0.15–0.20 g/kg) or placebo for 2 years. Primary outcome measures were the effect of treatment on clinical disability, measured by the change in EDSS, and the proportion of patients with improved, stable, or worse disability (at least 1 point on the EDSS scale). Intent-to-treat analysis showed that IVIG had a significant, albeit small, beneficial effect on the EDSS end points. In addition, it reduced relapse rates by about half without having an apparent effect on relapse severity. However, it is possible that blinding was not optimal, and this may have biased the study results. Unfortunately, MRI examinations were not obtained in this study and no data on 3-month or 6-month "confirmed" EDSS changes were presented.

In another study, involving 26 patients, an effect of higher doses of IVIG (2.0 g/kg monthly for 6 months) on MRI activity could be established, but in this study there were a high number of drop-outs because of adverse events.

In an Israeli double-blind study of 40 patients with RRMS, people were randomly assigned to receive a loading dose of IVIG (0.4 mg/kg/day for 5 days), followed by single boosters (0.4 mg/kg) or placebo once every 2 months for 2 years. Annual exacerbation rate was reduced by about 40 percent and there was an effect on EDSS scores. However, total lesion score on brain MRI did not show a significant difference between groups.

A recent phase three trial of IVIg in 318 patients with SPMS did not show any clinical benefit on relapse rate or disability progression.

Severe side effects of treatment with IVIG are uncommon, but can include thromboembolism, aseptic meningitis, renal failure, viral infection, eczema, and anaphylaxis. Another potential problem associated with the use of IVIG is that a number of studies have shown that the constituents present in commercially available IVIG preparations can be quite variable.

In addition to having immunoregulatory capacity (by suppressing production of pro-inflammatory cytokines or by containing anti-idiotypic antibodies), some studies suggest that IVIG might be able to promote remyelination. However, small clinical studies performed at the Mayo Clinic do not support the hypothesis that IVIG might be effective in reversing long-standing neurologic and visual deficits.

In the opinion of the Committee, the results of the studies that have been published are controversial. Results of further studies should be awaited before a clear recommendation can be made. Therefore, routine use of IVIG is not currently advised.

Azathioprine

Azathioprine is an immunosuppressive drug that is widely used in a variety of immune-mediated disorders. A meta-analysis of five double-blind and two single-blind, randomized, controlled trials involving a total of 793 MS patients supported the conclusion that oral azathioprine (1–3 mg/kg/m2) reduces the rate of relapse and might have a very small effect on EDSS scores. These results have been criticized on the basis that inadequate azathioprine doses were used in some of these trials. Another recent meta-analysis of published studies suggested that azathioprine may have a similar effect on 2-year probability of freedom from relapse to the interferons in reducing relapse rate. A number of trials are currently in progress to determine the potential treatment effects of azathioprine administered either alone or in combination with the interferons. Side effects include gastrointestinal, hematological, and hepatic toxicity. Another potential risk of long-term therapy is cancer, although a case-controlled study suggests that short-term use (less than 5 years) is not associated with a significantly increased risk. Careful monitoring of the patient (including blood cell counts and liver function tests) is necessary throughout the course of treatment.

In the opinion of the Committee, therapy with azathioprine has been demonstrated to have limited usefulness in selected patients. Although it is generally well tolerated, its use carries risk.

Cyclophosphamide

Cyclophosphamide is another immunosuppressive drug that has been used in MS treatment for many years. Its early use was mostly in uncontrolled studies in which it was often, but not always, reported to improve the condition of patients with chronic progressive MS, especially those with only modest disability at the beginning of treatment. The largest trial performed, a Canadian multicenter study, failed to demonstrate benefit. A number of incompletely blinded, uncontrolled studies continue to suggest that intensive immunosuppression with cyclophosphamide may reduce clinical and MRI evidence of aggressive disease activity in selected patients. Cyclophosphamide has many side effects, including hair loss, nausea and vomiting, hemorrhagic cystitis, infertility, and risk of infection. Some clinicians still use cyclophosphamide as a "booster" in rapidly progressive patients, based on reports that it may stabilize the disease. Careful monitoring of the patient, including blood cell counts, liver function tests, and urinalysis, is necessary throughout the course of treatment.

In the opinion of the Committee, there remains considerable controversy about the merits of this drug in MS in the absence of positive results from large, randomized, and controlled studies. Because its use carries significant risk, further use should be regarded as investigational.

Cyclosporin-A

Cyclosporin-A is an effective immunosuppressive agent that is chiefly responsible for improved success rates with kidney, heart, and liver transplants. It also has been found to be effective in some autoimmune diseases. It was studied in a number of clinical trials in MS, the largest involving 547 patients with chronic progressive disease. It was found to slightly reduce the progression rate and delay the time to requiring use of a wheelchair. These marginal to modest benefits from treatment, however, are outweighed by the long-term toxicity of the drug in impairing kidney function and causing hypertension.

In the opinion of the Committee, cyclosporin-A has some efficacy, but the association with serious side effects makes it an unsuitable therapy in MS.

Methotrexate

Methotrexate is another immunosuppressive agent. Low-dose oral administration has been shown to be both effective and relatively nontoxic in other immunologically mediated diseases, such as rheumatoid arthritis and psoriasis. An early trial in MS showed some reduction in the relapse rate but no benefit in patients with progressive disease.

In another study, 60 ambulatory patients with progressive MS and moderate to severe disability were treated with methotrexate in a dosage of 7.5 mg weekly or placebo for 2 years. Patients receiving active treatment showed significantly reduced worsening according to a composite measure of outcome that included the EDSS and tests of arm function, the maximal benefit occurring relatively early in the study. However, the effect of this treatment was not significant when a traditional outcome measure such as the EDSS was used. The effect on MRI activity also was marginal. This low dose of methotrexate was well tolerated, and none of the patients discontinued treatment because of side effects. Several small studies have been published indicating that methotrexate, when added to one of the interferons, may reduce disease activity, but these reports are not definitive.

Prolonged use of methotrexate may cause mucosal irritation, gastrointestinal symptoms, hepatotoxicity, pulmonary fibrosis, and bone marrow suppression.

In the opinion of the Committee, the benefit of methotrexate has not been proven, and further studies are needed. Low-dose therapy seems to be well tolerated.

Cladribine (2-Chlorodeoxyadenosine)

Cladribine is an immunosuppressive drug that produces a phenomenon of relatively selective lymphocyte killing (apoptosis) because of a resistance of the effects of adenosine deaminase. It was tested in MS patients and has a background in the treatment of lymphoid neoplasms and other autoimmune disorders.

The first-year results of a double-blind, placebo-controlled, cross-over study of intravenous cladribine in 50 patients with progressive MS, which was designed as a 2-year study, were favorable. Neurologic scores and total lesion volumes on MRI were stable or improved in the patients receiving cladribine, but continued to deteriorate in patients on placebo. These favorable results could not be replicated in a recent phase III study in which 159 patients with progressive MS were randomized to receive cladribine in two different doses (0.7 or 2.1 mg/kg) or placebo. Patients were assessed monthly for 12 months with serial evaluation of disability scores and semiannual measurement of MRI. Although cladribine treatment had a remarkable effect in reducing the volume of gadolinium enhancement on MRI, a significant effect on disability could not be shown. The side-effect profile of this compound includes bone marrow suppression and increased susceptibility to viral infections (especially herpes zoster). Studies with oral cladribine are being planned.

In the opinion of the Committee, therapy with cladribine has no proven clinical benefit. It must be considered investigational at this time because its use carries significant risk.

Sulfasalazine

Sulfasalazine is a well-established, safe drug with known anti-inflammatory and immunomodulatory properties. It has been used as a treatment for inflammatory bowel disease for a number of decades. More recently, it also proved to have a favorable impact on rheumatoid arthritis. The results of a large Mayo Clinic–Canadian cooperative, double-blind, placebo-controlled, phase III trial of sulfasalazine in active MS have been reported. A total of 199 ambulatory MS patients with active disease were treated with sulfasalazine up to 2 grams a day or placebo and were evaluated for a minimum of 3 years (mean follow-up 3.7 years). Even though the short-term (2-year) response seemed to be favorable, the drug ultimately failed to slow or prevent disability progression as measured by the primary outcome (confirmed worsening of the EDSS score by at least 1 point on two consecutive 3-month visits).

In the opinion of the Committee, sulfasalazine does not have benefit in MS.

Interferon Alpha

Interferon alpha is, like IFN beta, a type 1 IFN (see section on IFN beta for explanation). They both use the same receptor, and therefore it is plausible that IFN alpha might also have a favorable impact on the course of MS.

The first large trial of recombinant IFN alpha studied 98 patients for 1 year in a double-blind, randomized, placebo-controlled manner; this trial showed no clear benefit. More recently, a 6-month study of 20 patients was done in Italy with MRI monitoring. New or enlarging lesions occurred more often in scans of placebo-treated patients, and IFN alpha–treated patients had fewer exacerbations. The latter study used higher doses of IFN alpha than had been used in earlier trials, given by every-other-day intramuscular injection.

In the opinion of the Committee, the rationale of IFN alpha therapy is plausible and the treatment might well be effective, but larger trials are necessary to establish its safety and efficacy.

Corticosteroids

Chronic treatment with glucocorticoids has failed to demonstrate a beneficial effect on either the progression of disability or the rate of relapse. In addition, it may induce severe adverse effects, including osteoporosis, aseptic bone necrosis, proximal muscle weakness, hypertension, hyperglycemia, cataracts, and psychiatric events. One recent randomized trial found that patients who received regularly scheduled corticosteroid treatments (1 g IV methylprednisolone for 5 days, followed by 4 days of prednisone [50 mg and 25 mg for 2 days, each] every 4 months for 3 years, and then twice yearly for 2 years) were less likely to develop MRI evidence of brain atrophy, clinical evidence of progressive disability, or convert from relapsing to SPMS than were patients treated "as needed" with corticosteroids. This study is of potential interest but has not been confirmed to date.

> *In the opinion of the Committee, chronic therapy with corticosteroids is contraindicated in MS because of lack of efficacy and reported harmful effects (for pulse treatment with steroids see Chapter 2).*

Interferon Gamma

> *In the opinion of the Committee, therapy with interferon gamma is contraindicated in MS because of reported harmful effects (see section on interferon beta on page 24).*

Plasmapheresis

In a large, multicenter, placebo-controlled, Canadian study, the value of chronic plasmapheresis (PE) could not be proven. In this study, conducted over a 2-year period, PE in association with oral cyclophosphamide and prednisone did not prevent progression of MS disability any more than placebo and sham PE. As discussed in Chapter 2, plasmapheresis may "rescue" (e.g., induce significant clinical improvement) up to 40 percent of relapsed MS and neuromyelitis optica patients who have failed to improve following treatment with high dose corticosteroids in the setting of a recent attack.

> *In the opinion of the Committee, the rationale behind plasmapheresis is plausible, but it has not been exten-*

sively tested so far, and therefore must be regarded as experimental.

Acyclovir (Zovirax®) and Other Antiviral Agents

There still is the possibility that viruses play an important role in the etiopathogenesis of MS. Therefore, a randomized, double-blind study of acyclovir, an agent commonly used for the treatment of herpes simplex infections, was performed. Sixty patients with RRMS were treated with acyclovir 800 mg three times a day or placebo. A 34 percent reduction in the annual relapse rate was reported during active treatment, warranting further research of acyclovir and related agents. A recent trial of valacyclovir failed to demonstrate benefit in RRMS.

In the opinion of the Committee, the rationale behind antiviral therapy is partly plausible, but it has not been extensively tested so far, and therefore must be regarded as experimental.

Bone Marrow Transplantation and Hemopoietic Stem Cell Transplantation

Bone marrow transplantation (BMT) is widely used in a number of neoplastic diseases, and there have been a number of reports suggesting that it may also be beneficial in several autoimmune diseases. The procedure consists of a severe immunosuppressive regimen provided by high-dose chemotherapy or total body irradiation followed by IV infusion (transplantation) of bone marrow-derived hematopoietic stem cells. During the first months after BMT, transplant recipients are exposed to many sources of complications, some of which are potentially lethal. The procedure has been shown to be effective in EAE, and there are anecdotal (poorly documented) reports of therapeutic efficacy in MS. The European Study Group for Blood and Marrow Transplantation is in the process of developing guidelines to define criteria for patient selection and transplantation procedures for studies to be initiated in the near future.

In the opinion of the Committee, the rationale of BMT is plausible and warrants investigation in well-designed studies carried out in centers with experience in managing profoundly immunocompromised patients. BMT carries serious risk.

EMERGING TREATMENTS: ALEMTUZUMAB, STATINS, ESTRIOL, AND OTHERS

Alemtuzumab

Alemtuzumab (Campath®) is a humanized anti-leukocyte monoclonal antibody. In patients with SPMS, it has been shown to induce pronounced effects on the immune system as well as marked suppression of cerebral inflammation, as documented on serial MRIs. In addition, there has been a suppression of relapses. There are concerns with respect to the safety of the compound because in these early studies about 30 percent of patients developed Graves' disease, an autoimmune thyroid condition. A recently initiated clinical trial will compare safety and efficacy of two doses of alemtuzumab with a standard treatment of interferon beta-1a (Rebif®) in patients with early, active RRMS.

Statins

Statins are orally-administered, lipid-lowering drugs. Statins have already been shown to ameliorate clinical signs in EAE, an animal model for MS. Furthermore, *in vitro* data demonstrate that these agents have several potentially favorable immunomodulatory actions that make them candidate treatments for MS.

Recently, 30 individuals with RRMS, who had at least one new lesion during a 3-month screening period involving monthly

MRIs, were treated with a very high dose (80 mg) of simvastatin (Zocor®) daily. Preliminary analysis of the results indicates a significant (43 percent) decrease in the mean number of new lesions on monthly MRI during months 4, 5, and 6 of the treatment period, and in the volume of new lesions. Due to the limitations of the study design (small number of patients, no placebo controls, and inclusion on the basis of baseline activity, thus probably selecting for subsequent regression to the mean) these results should be interpreted with caution.

Among potential future therapies for MS, statins are especially interesting because they are given orally and have an outstanding safety record. The main question is whether effective immunomodulation occurs at the cholesterol-lowering doses currently used clinically. Additional studies are planned.

Estriol

Following the observation that MS patients are less likely to have relapses during pregnancy, a small, open-label study of daily high-dose (8 mg/day) estriol was recently published showing an apparent reduction in MRI evidence of disease activity in the six RRMS patients but not in the six SPMS patients. Again, further work is needed in this area. Potential benefits of estriol, when given for long periods, have to be weighed against side-effects and toxicity, including risks for carcinogenesis and thrombosis.

Other Experimental Treatments

The aim of several experimental therapies is to modulate the specific immune response in some way or another. One way would be to induce antigen-specific tolerance by modifying the method of applying the antigen; for example, via the gut ("oral tolerance"). Unfortunately, however, in MS the oral administration of myelin has been ineffective, despite encouraging results in a small pilot study. A problem for this approach, of course, is that a MS-specific antigen so far has not been identified.

T cell (receptor) vaccination is another method that is being applied in clinical trials. The concept is that injection of disease-causing T cells, or their specific T cell receptors, isolated from a recipient and undergoing culturing and inactivation, as a vaccine stimulates regulatory mechanisms. Some promising immunological responses have been observed in small studies, but so far rigorous proof of efficacy is still lacking.

Future studies will also include the administration of neuro-protective agents or molecules that would facilitate axonal re-growth, the administration of growth factors that promote the proliferation and survival of oligodendrocytes, the cells that make myelin, and the transplantation of cells (e.g., neural stem cells or progenitor cells) that are capable of making new myelin.

In the opinion of the Committee, the approaches mentioned in this "Emerging Treatments" section require more research before their role in the treatment of MS can be determined. At this time their use cannot be recommended outside the context of well-designed clinical trials.

Although proof has become available that we have developed the tools to generate intervention strategies that are effective in the treatment of patients with MS, we must be careful that in this atmosphere of optimism we do not too easily adopt new therapeutic approaches based on the results of small studies without phase III trials involving large numbers of patients being performed. There is increasing pressure towards shorter studies to obtain quick answers, even though it has been observed that short-term favorable trends may reverse with prolonged follow-up; for example, an immunomodulatory agent (Linomide®) that had shown promising effects in phase II studies had to be withdrawn from phase III studies because of unexpected serious (cardiovascular) side effects.

In a disease such as MS, in which disability generally accumulates slowly over many years, severe side effects, even if infrequent, might invalidate a therapeutic approach.

Even with the development of MRI as a more and more powerful tool to study therapeutic interventions, there is a need to obtain meaningful, robust data on long-term clinical efficacy and safety. There is still no substitute for longer-term, carefully monitored, randomized clinical trials. In addition to generating the registration data required for regulatory approval, clinical trials should also be seen as instruments to test research hypotheses on mechanism of action and the type of patients to respond most favorably. As evidence mounts that MS comprises several distinct subforms, the choice of treatment for individual patients, ideally, should be determined by knowledge of the specific underlying pathophysiologic mechanism and the respective profile of available drugs. The ultimate goal is tailor-made therapy.

Guide for Further Reading

Interferon Beta

- Cohen JA, Cutter GR, Fischer JS, Goodman Ad, Heidenreich FR, Kooijman MF, et al. Benefit of interferon â-1a on MSFC progression in secondary progressive MS. *Neurology* 2002; 59:679–687.

- Comi G, Filippi M, Barkhof F, et al. Effect of early interferon treatment on conversion to definite multiple sclerosis: a randomized study. *Lancet* 2001; (357)9268: 1576–82.

- Durelli L, Verdun E, Barbero P, et al. Every-other-day interferon beta-1b versus once-weekly interferon beta-1a for multiple sclerosis: results of a 2-year prospective randomized multicentre study (INCOMIN). *Lancet* 2002; (359)9316:1453–60.

- European Study Group on interferon beta-1b in secondary progressive MS. Placebo-controlled multicentre randomized trial of interferon beta-1b in treatment of secondary progressive multiple sclerosis. *Lancet* 1998; 352: 1491–1497.

- Filippini G, Munari L, Incorvaia B, Ebers GC, Polman C, D'Amico R, et al. Interferons in relapsing remitting multiple sclerosis: a systematic review. *Lancet* 2003; 361:545–552.

- Jacobs LD, Beck RW, Simon JH, Kindel RP, Brownscheidle CM, Murray TJ, et al. Intramuscular interferon beta-1a therapy initiated during a first demyelinating event in multiple sclerosis. *N Engl J Med* 2000; 343:898–904.

- Jacobs LD, Cookfair DL, Rudick RA, et al. Intramuscular interferon beta-1a for disease progression in relapsing multiple sclerosis. *Ann Neurol* 1996; 39:285–294.

- Leary SM, Miller DH, Stevenson VL, Brex PA, Chard DT, Thompson AJ. Interferon beta-1a in primary progressive MS. An exploratory, randomized, controlled trial. *Neurology* 2003; 60:44–51.

- Li DKB, Paty DW, UBC MS/MRI Analysis Research Group, and the PRISMS Study Group. Magnetic resonance imaging results of the PRIS*MS trial: A randomized, double-blind, placebo-controlled study of interferon beta-1a in relapsing remitting multiple sclerosis. *Ann Neurol* 1999; 46:197–206.

- Miller DH, Molyneux PD, Barker GJ, et al. Effect of interferon beta-1b on magnetic resonance imaging outcomes in secondary progressive multiple sclerosis: Results of a European multicenter randomized double-blind placebo-controlled trial. *Ann Neurol* 1999; 46:850–859.

- North American Study Group on Interferon beta-1b in Secondary Progressive MS: results from a three-year controlled study. *Neurology* 2004; 63:1788–1795.

- Panitch H, Goodin DS, Francis G, et al. Randomized, comparative study of interferon beta-1a treatment regimens in MS: The EVIDENCE Trial. [comment]. *Neurology* 2002; (59)10:1496–506.

- Paty DW, Li DKB, the UBC MS/MRI Study Group, and the IFNB Multiple Sclerosis Study Group. Interferon beta-1b is effective in relapsing remitting multiple sclerosis. II. MRI analysis. *Neurology* 1993; 43:662–667.

- PRISMS Study Group. Randomized, double-blind placebo-controlled study of interferon beta-1a in relapsing remitting multiple sclerosis. *Lancet* 1998; 352:1498–1504.

- Rudick RA, Goodkin DE, Jacobs LD, et al. The impact of interferon beta-1a on neurologic disability in multiple sclerosis. *Neurology* 1997; 49:358–363.

- Secondary Progressive Efficacy Clinical Trial of Recombinant Interferon-beta-1a in MS Study Group. Randomized controlled trial of interferon-beta-1a in secondary progressive MS—Clinical results. *Neurology* 2001; (56)11:1496–1504.

- Simon JH, Jacobs LD, Campion M, et al. Magnetic resonance studies of intramuscular interferon beta-1a for relapsing multiple sclerosis. *Ann Neurol* 1998; 43:79–87.

- Sorensen PS, Ross C, Clemmesen K, et al. Clinical importance of neutralising antibodies against interferon beta in patients with relapsing-remitting multiple sclerosis. *Lancet* 2003; (362):1184–1191.

- The IFNB Multiple Sclerosis Study Group. Interferon beta-1b is effective in relapsing remitting multiple sclerosis. I. Clinical results. *Neurology* 1993; 43:655–661.

Glatiramer Acetate

- Comi G, Filippi M, Wolinsky JS. European/Canadian multicenter, double-blind, randomized, placebo-controlled study of the effects of glatiramer acetate on magnetic resonance imaging–measured disease activity and burden in patients with relapsing multiple sclerosis. European/Canadian Glatiramer Acetate Study Group. *Ann Neurol* 2001; (49)3: 290–7.

- Johnson KP, Brooks BR, Cohen JA, et al. Copolymer 1 reduces relapse rate and improves disability in relapsing-remitting multiple sclerosis: Results of a phase III multicenter, double-blind, placebo-controlled trial. *Neurology* 1995; 45:1268–1276.

- Johnson KP, Brooks BR, Cohen JA, et al. Extended use of glatiramer acetate (Copaxone) is well tolerated and maintains its clinical effect on multiple sclerosis relapse rate and degree of disability. *Neurology* 1998; 50: 701–708.

Natalizumab

- For phase III trials, see Web site: www.FDA.com.

- Miller DH, Khan OR, Sheremata WA, Blumhardt LD, Rice GPA, Libonati MA, et al. A controlled trial of Natalizumab for relapsing multiple sclerosis. *N Engl J Med* 2003; 348:15–23.

Intravenous Immunoglobulin

- Fazekas F, Deisenhammer F, Strasser-Fuchs S, et al. Randomized placebo-controlled trial of monthly intravenous immunoglobulin therapy in relapsing remitting multiple sclerosis. *Lancet* 1997; 349:589–593.

- Hommes OR, Sorensen PS, Fazekas F, et al. Intravenous immunoglobulin in secondary progressive multiple sclerosis: randomized placebo-controlled trial. *Lancet* 2004; 364:1149–1156.

- Sorensen PS, Wanscher B, Jensen CV, et al. Intravenous immunoglobulin G reduces MRI activity in relapsing multiple sclerosis. *Neurology* 1998; 50:1273–1281.

Mitoxantrone

- Edan G, Miller D, Clanet M, et al. Therapeutic effect of mitoxantrone combined with methylprednisolone in multiple sclerosis: A randomized multicentre study of active disease using MRI and clinical criteria. *J Neurol Neurosurg Psychiatry* 1997; 62:112–118.

- Hartung HP, Gonsette R, Koenig N, et al. Mitoxantrone in progressive multiple sclerosis: a placebo-controlled, double-blind, randomized, multicentre trial. *Lancet* 2002; 360:2018–25.

- Millefiorini E, Gasperini C, Pozzilli C, et al. Randomized placebo-controlled trial of mitoxantrone in relapsing-remitting multiple sclerosis: A 24-month clinical and MRI outcome. *J Neurol* 1997; 244:153–159.

Other Immunosuppressive Agents

- Goodkin DE, Rudick RA, VanderBrug, Medendorp S, et al. Low-dose (7.5 mg) oral methotrexate reduces the rate of progression in chronic progressive multiple sclerosis. *Ann Neurol* 1995; 37:30–40.

- Palace J, Rothwell P. New treatments and azathioprine in multiple sclerosis. [comment]. *Lancet* 1997; (350) 9073:261.

- Rice GPA for the Cladribine Clinical Study Group; and Filippi M and Comi GC for the Cladribine MRI Study Group. Cladribine and progressive MS: Clinical and MRI outcomes of a multicenter controlled trial. *Neurology* 2000; 54:1145–1155.

Plasmapheresis

- Keegan M, Pineda AA, McClelland RL, et al. Plasma exchange for severe attacks of CNS demyelination: predictors of response. *Neurology* 2002; (58):143–146.

- Weinshenker BG, O'Brien PC, Petterson TM, et al. A randomized trial of plasma exchange in acute central nervous system inflammatory demyelinating disease. *Ann Neurol* 1999; 46:878–886.

Bone Marrow Transplantation

- Comi G, Kappos L, Clanet M, et al. Guidelines for autologous blood and marrow stem cell transplantation in multiple sclerosis: a consensus report written on behalf of the European Group for Blood and Marrow Transplantation and the European Charcot Foundation. BMT-MS Study Group. *J Neurol* 2000; (247)5:376–82.

- Saiz A, Blanco Y, Carreras E, et al. Clinical and MRI outcome after autologous hematopoietic stem cell transplantation in MS. *Neurology* 2004; (62)2:282–284.

Antiviral Treatment

- Bech E, Lycke J, Gadeberg P, et al. A randomized, double-blind, placebo-controlled MRI study of anti-herpes virus therapy in MS. [see comment] [summary for patients in *Curr Neurol Neurosci Rep*. 2002 May; 2(3):257–8; PMID:11937004]. *Neurology* (58)1:31–6.

Emerging Treatments

- Hohlfeld R, Wekerle H. Autoimmune concepts of multiple sclerosis as a basis for selective immunotherapy: From pipe dreams to (therapeutic) pipelines. *PNAS* 2004; 101:14599–14606.

- Miller DH, Khan OA, Sheremata WA, Blumhardt LD, Rice GPA, Libonati MA, et al. A controlled trial of Natalizumab for relapsing multiple sclerosis. *N Engl J Med* 2003; 348:15–23.

- Sicotte NL, Liva SM, Klutch R, et al. Treatment of multiple sclerosis with the pregnancy hormone estriol. *Ann Neurol*. 2002 (52)4:421–8.

- Vollmer T, Key L, Durkalski V, et al. Oral simvastatin treatment in relapsing-remitting multiple sclerosis. [see comment]. *Lancet* 2004; (363)9421:1607–8.

Chapter 4

Symptomatic Treatment, Neurorehabilitation, and Service Delivery

Multiple sclerosis involves multiple areas of the central nervous system and therefore can produce a diverse range of symptoms, from visual loss to pain, fatigue, and paraparesis. In the initial stages of the condition, the symptoms are often isolated, relating to a single area of inflammation, although multiple areas may be involved (e.g., optic nerve and spinal cord). Symptoms usually are transient, but even in these early stages recovery may be less than complete, leaving residual disturbance, which is either constant or reemerges with exercise (e.g., Uhthoff's phenomenon). There are some people in whom the initial presentation, usually a mild spastic paraparesis (spasticity and weakness that leads to difficulty in walking), progressively worsens without any remission (primary progressive MS [PPMS]).

In time, the majority of patients develop an increasing range of symptoms, many of which worsen slowly and result in progressive and complex disability. This poses particular problems in terms of management, in that the symptoms tend to interact with each other, and it may be inappropriate to treat one symptom in isolation. For example, the carrying out of clean, intermittent self-catheterization to manage bladder control must take into account the patient's cognitive ability, upper limb dexterity, and lower limb mobility (in relation to spasticity, etc.). It is also important to appreciate that the treatment of one symptom may worsen another, such as the effects of antispasticity or antidepressant agents in people already suffering from severe fatigue. This is, at least in part, the rationale behind the need for goal-orientated multidisciplinary rehabilitation.

This chapter discusses the treatment of individual symptoms followed by rehabilitation and service provision. In contrast to the previous section, which was able to call upon evidence from randomized control trials, there is a paucity of such data available in symptomatic management and rehabilitation. The studies that have been carried out have tended to be small and poorly designed. To address this deficit, two important initiatives were set up—the Multiple Sclerosis Council for Clinical Practice Guidelines (MSCCPG) (which has since been disbanded) and the establishment of the Cochrane Collaboration for Multiple Sclerosis.

The MSCCPG was a collaboration of a number of key organizations involved in MS, including the Consortium of Multiple Sclerosis Centers (North America), Rehabilitation in Multiple Sclerosis (RIMS – A European Organization of MS Centers), and the Multiple Sclerosis International Federation (MSIF). The MSCCPG has published guidelines on fatigue, bladder management, and spasticity. The Cochrane Collaboration is applying the principle of evaluating randomized controlled trials to look at aspects of the management of MS. In relation to symptomatic management, current protocols include the role of the aminopyridines in MS, the treatment of spasticity, and pain management.

In the United Kingdom, the National Institute for Clinical Excellence has produced detailed guidance on the management of MS, incorporating all available supporting evidence, which is a valuable resource (NICE 2003 – www.nice.org.uk).

SYMPTOMATIC TREATMENT OF MS

The treatment of individual symptoms is discussed in this section, bearing in mind that the majority of people have multiple symptoms that interact in a complex and disabling fashion. For example, poor mobility may result from any or all of the following impairments: lower limb and truncal weakness, spasticity, cerebellar ataxia, reduced sensory input, and visual symptoms. Similarly, fatigue, mood disturbance, and cognitive dysfunction also interact and may complicate both evaluation and subsequent management. Even when considering individual symptoms, it is essential to appreciate that drug treatment is of limited value but often is optimally used in association with therapy. For example, spasticity can rarely be managed by oral agents alone, but it may be greatly helped by a combination of education, physical therapy and medication. Patient education is particularly important in the management of symptoms such as spasticity, in which basic practical issues such as posture, standing program, and so forth are crucial, but it applies equally to most, if not all, other symptoms such as ataxia, fatigue, and pain.

Spasticity

Spasticity is a frequent symptom in MS that is seen to a greater or lesser extent in up to 75 percent of patients. It is a complex, poorly understood symptom that is often associated with muscle weakness. In MS, the lower limbs are more markedly affected by spasticity than the arms. Spasticity may be associated with pain, painful extensor and flexor spasms, clonus, and underlying weakness. Extensor spasticity of the legs, particularly of the quadriceps, might be considered advantageous for standing, walking, and transferring. However, sudden loss of tone may also occur when the muscle reaches a certain crucial length as a result of increasing resistance and progressive stretching. Spasticity is associated with structural changes in the muscles (thixotropy) leading to further resistance to movement and shortening. Functionally, spasticity can reduce mobility and dexterity; spasms may prevent transfers, hinder comfortable sitting and lying postures, and affect sleep.

The treatment of spasticity should not be aimed at its removal per se, but rather at improving function, easing care, or alleviating pain. Key components in the management of spasticity include patient education, physiotherapy input, and the judicious use of drug treatment. This should include awareness that noxious stimuli, such as urinary tract infections, bowel impaction, and ingrown toenails, may worsen spasticity. The importance of correct positioning in lying and sitting, and the value of a standing program should be emphasized. Treatment may be divided into oral therapy, drugs given by other routes (intrathecal, intraneural, or intramuscular), and surgery. It must be remembered that whatever treatment is chosen, expert monitoring is required. Furthermore, MS-related spasticity tends to change over time, and it is important to reevaluate treatments at regular intervals.

There are few trials of antispasticity agents in MS. However, they usually involve small numbers of patients in which the pattern of spasticity is inadequately described, the objectives of treatment are not specified, and only short- to medium-term outcomes are assessed. In clinical practice it is suggested that only one substance be used at a time, although there may be a rationale for combining drugs if a single agent is ineffective or only partially effective. Of the available agents, baclofen has undergone the most evaluation (both the oral and intrathecal routes). Tizanidine has been the most recently licensed drug in the United Kingdom and the United States. Most of the studies were carried out 20 to 30 years ago, and many focused on spinal cord injury. The management of severe spasticity may be best provided by a multidisciplinary clinic that incorporates neurologic, physiologic, and physiotherapy expertise, and can provide a wide range of treatment options.

Oral Agents for Spasticity

Baclofen.   This g-aminobutyric acid (GABA)-B receptor agonist acts mainly on the presynaptic and postsynaptic terminals of primary fibers of the spinal cord to reduce the release of amino acids and to antagonize their actions. It is particularly useful in the treatment of painful spasms and increased tone of spinal origin, although functional benefits have been more difficult to demonstrate. In a large study of 759 patients with MS, 70 percent showed marked improvement in spasticity (defined as a two-step reduction on the five-step Ashworth Scale) and flexor spasms. A beneficial effect on spasms and hypertonicity was also seen in a small, double-blind, placebo-controlled, crossover study that involved 22 patients, 11 of whom had MS. The efficacy of baclofen has been shown to be equal to, if not greater than, that of diazepam. Baclofen is given three times a day, and should be started at a very low level with gradually increasing steps of 5 to 10 mg until the desired effect is achieved and/or side effects such as drowsiness, fatigue, and muscle weakness become unacceptable, usually reaching a dose of between 40–80 mg a day. Side effects are reported to affect up to 45 percent of patients. Abrupt discontinuation may result in severe withdrawal symptoms, which include hallucinations and seizures.

Tizanidine.   This imidazoline derivative, which is closely related to clonidine, acts by stimulating b2-adrenergic receptors in the spinal cord. A number of studies have suggested that its efficacy is similar to that of baclofen. More recently, it was evaluated in two double-blind, placebo-controlled trials in the United Kingdom and the United States involving 187 and 220 patients, respectively. In the American trial, tizanidine reduced spasms and clonus significantly, but had no effect on spasticity as measured on the Ashworth Scale, and although the patients rated the drug significantly better on efficacy, the assessing physician did not. In the UK trial, a 20 percent reduction in spasticity was reported, and 75 percent of patients receiving the drug reported a subjective benefit without an increase in muscle weakness. However, no improvement in mobility-related activities of daily living was found. The suggestion that it may not cause weakness may be of therapeutic value. It is suggested that it be started at a low dose, 2 mg three times a day, and gradually increased up to a maximum of between 18–36 mgs. A long-acting preparation that may be taken once daily is available in some countries. The most frequent side effects are tiredness (a major problem in patients who already suffer from fatigue), drowsiness, and dry mouth. Liver function tests must be checked before and after treatment because hepatotoxicity may occur.

Dantrolene.   Few studies have evaluated the role of this agent or its efficacy in the management of spasticity. However, because dantrolene has a peripheral target of action and exerts its effect within the muscle itself by inhibiting the release of calcium ions from the sarcoplasmic reticulum, thereby preventing muscle contraction, it is theoretically a useful additional agent if centrally acting drugs are not effective. It is thought to be more effective in treating spasms and clonus than hypertonicity, and long-term benefit has been documented. However, it is poorly tolerated. Side effects include drowsiness, weakness, fatigue, and occasionally hepatotoxicity, which may be irreversible.

Benzodiazepines.   Benzodiazepines have three potential anti-spasticity actions: suppression of sensory impulses from muscle and skin receptors, potentiation of GABA action post-synaptically, and inhibition of excitatory descending pathways. The efficacy of diazepam has been evaluated in a small, double-blind, cross-over trial of 21 patients with spastic paraparesis. It may be used as additional therapy in resistant cases of spasticity. Its role is limited by side effects, including drowsiness and dependence.

Cannabinoids.   (See also Chapter 5.) There has been increasing pressure to evaluate the role of cannabinoids in spasticity in MS. A recent study evaluated the potential benefit of cannabinoids on spasticity and other symptoms related to MS. It was a random-ized, placebo-controlled trial that enrolled 667 patients with stable MS and muscle spasticity; 630 participants were treated at 33 UK centers with oral cannabis extract (n=211), Delta9-tetrahydrocannabinol (Delta9-THC; n=206), or placebo (n=213). The trial duration was 15 weeks. The primary outcome measure was change in overall spasticity as measured by the Ashworth scale. Analysis was by intention to treat; 611 of 630 patients were followed up for the primary endpoint. No treatment effect of cannabinoids on the primary outcome was seen (p=0.40). The estimated difference in mean reduction in total Ashworth score for participants taking cannabis extract compared with placebo was 0.32 (95 percent CI −1.04 to 1.67), and for those taking Delta9-THC versus placebo it was 0.94 (−0.44 to 2.31). A treat-ment effect on patient-reported spasticity and pain was seen (p=0.003), and patients reported improvement in spasticity in 61 percent, 60 percent, and 46 percent of participants on cannabis extract, Delta9-THC, and placebo, respectively. However, the study showed evidence of a placebo effect, and there was also an element of patient un-blinding.

A 12-month follow-up, which included data on 502 patients, was subsequently reported. There was evidence of a treatment effect on muscle spasticity as measured by change in Ashworth score from baseline to 12-months follow-up in an intention to treat analysis, (p=0.04). In the group taking Delta9-THC, the Ashworth score was significantly reduced compared to those taking either cannabis extract or placebo.

Another, smaller study carried out in a rehabilitation setting failed to show an objective benefit on spasticity, and an earlier, double-blind, placebo-controlled, twofold, crossover trial of oral *tetrahydrocannabinol* (THC) and *Cannabis sativa* plant extract in 16 patients showed no benefit, and both treatments worsened the global impression of the patients. Thus, the current evidence evaluating the use of cannabinoids in the treatment of spasticity in MS is variable, and may relate in part to the poor respon-siveness of the outcome measure and the difficulty in blinding.

Further research into cannabinoids is warranted and is currently underway

Other Drugs. A range of other drugs has been tried in MS-related spasticity, and reports involving small numbers have appeared in the literature. These drugs include clonazepam, memantine, glycine, L-threonine, vigabatrin, and, more recently, gabapentin.

Other Routes of Administration in Spasticity

In very severe spasticity, high doses of oral agents are likely to be either ineffective or not tolerated, and drugs may best be given intrathecally via a subcutaneously placed infusion pump. Although this is an invasive treatment, it is very efficient. Less than one hundredth of the oral dose is required to achieve the required effect. The intrathecal route was originally described for the use of phenol, but more recently it has been evaluated for baclofen. Dramatic effects on tone (as measured by the Ashworth Scale) and spasm frequency were seen in MS and spinal cord injury. Some effect on function, particularly relating to transfers and self-care, has also been reported, but few investigators have evaluated the potential effect on quality of life. In this treatment, the effect is initially tested by bolus injection of 25 to 100 mcg given via a lumbar puncture before considering continuous drug application through an electronically programmed drug delivery system. Long-term treatment using *intrathecal baclofen* (ITB) has been evaluated and found to be beneficial. The main complications are technical and include pump malfunction, catheter-related problems (kinking, breaking, and displacement), local inflammation, and, rarely, spinal meningitis. Although the original studies were restricted to patients who were wheelchair users, ITB is now being used with encouraging results in more ambulatory patients. It should be used as part of a goal-orientated rehabilitation program, and careful assessment and selection is essential.

There has been a resurgence of interest in intrathecal phenol, which may be useful in improving care and posture in severely disabled patients who no longer have bowel and bladder function, and in whom sensation in the lower limbs is absent. In a recent retrospective study audit of 25 patients, benefit was seen in all patients, which translated into functional gains in most. Local treatment for more focal spasticity, with either nerve route injection with phenol and other agents, or muscle injection with botulinum toxin, is also used, although again there are few studies available for their evaluation. Large amounts of botulinum toxin are required and injections often need to be repeated every 3 to 6 months. A recent double-blind, placebo-controlled, dose-ranging study evaluated the role of botulinum toxin (Dysport® 500, 1000, 1500 units) in 74 MS patients with severe adductor spasticity. Range of hip movement and tone were improved in the treated groups, but all four groups had reduced spasms, showing improvement on a global rating scale. Only the 1000 and 1500 unit groups had improved hygiene scores, and the latter had the highest incidence of side effects. In general, however, botulinum toxin is considered to be more useful in the treatment of distal muscles in the arms and legs, and many practitioners are discouraged by the frequent large doses required for proximal lower limb spasticity in MS.

Surgery for Spasticity

Although a range of neurosurgical procedures is available for the management of spasticity, none have gained acceptance in the context of MS. There are relatively few data available to evaluate potential benefit, but some retrospective analyses of clinical series suggest that at least selective posterior rhizotomy may have a role.

In the view of the Committee, spasticity is a very disabling symptom that often is poorly managed. There is a range of treatment options that have a moderate evidence base, although none have shown absolute or comparative efficacy in a recent Cochrane review. However, a coordinated approach to management is essential, and there is a need for more effective oral agents with a better side-effect profile.

Ataxia and Tremor

Ataxia may be defined as a lack of or reduction in coordination and is invariably associated with tremor (i.e., an involuntary, rhythmic, oscillatory movement of a body part). These symptoms occur in 75 percent of patients with MS and most frequently manifest as upper limb intention tremor. They are both severely disabling and embarrassing, affecting upper limb function, gait, and, in severe cases of truncal ataxia, standing and sitting balance are badly affected. The tremor of MS is frequently only one component of a complex movement disorder and the underlying mechanisms are poorly understood. Although inflammatory demyelination in different parts of the cerebellum and related areas may produce a distinct tremor, it is nonetheless extremely difficult to classify individual tremors in patients. It remains one of the most difficult symptoms to manage and is associated with a poor outcome in rehabilitation.

As with spasticity, there are practical components to the management of ataxia, which must be considered before other interventions. These include patient education, improving posture, and maximizing proximal stability during activities, and the provision of equipment. Weights have not proved to be very successful, although they may be slightly more effective if a computer damping device is incorporated. A small exploratory study of occupational therapy input suggested modest benefit. Other treatments may include drug therapy, which is limited and often not well tolerated, and more invasive surgical intervention, including thalamotomy and thalamic stimulation.

Medical Treatment for Ataxia and Tremor

Few drugs have been evaluated and none adequately. Isoniazid (with pyridoxine) has been shown to be of limited benefit in a number of small studies. It showed some effect in 10 of 13 patients, although this did not translate into improved function. Four of six patients in a second study showed sufficient benefit that they wished to continue the drug. It is thought to be more useful in postural tremor with an intention component than in pure intention tremor. Up to 1200 mg a day in divided doses has been used, increasing gradually from 200 mg twice a day. This drug, which was the first to undergo a randomized control trial for the treatment of MS, is not well tolerated and causes gastrointestinal disturbance. There has been even less evaluation of other drugs, including carbamazepine, clonazepam, and buspirone. Propranolol may useful but higher doses, which may be poorly tolerated, are often required. Although a single-blind, cross-sectional study evaluating the role of carbamazepine in cerebellar tremor in 10 patients (7 with MS) suggested some benefit, it has also been suggested that this agent worsened ataxia. More recently, the 5-HT3 antagonist ondansetron has been evaluated, given by both intravenous and oral routes. Although the studies of the former looked promising, the more recent placebo-controlled, double-blind, parallel-group study of oral therapy was negative. Fifty-two patients, the majority of whom had MS, were randomized, and the treatment arm received 8 mg per day for 1 week. Although some benefit in the nine-hole peg test was seen in the treated arm, there was no difference between the groups on a global ataxia rating scale. A small study of cannabinoids in the treatment of ataxia failed to show any beneficial effect.

Surgical Intervention in Ataxia and Tremor

Although thalamotomy of the ventral intermediate nucleus (VIN) has been shown to be beneficial in the tremor of Parkinson's disease, there has been limited evaluation of its role in tremor relating to MS. In general, it is not considered to be as effective in this condition. In selected patients with MS, thalamotomy has been reported to alleviate contralateral limb tremor, initially in approximately 65 to 96 percent of cases, although in about 20 percent tremor returns within 12 months. Functional improvement is estimated to occur in 25 to 75 percent of patients. A recent study of unilateral thalamotomy compared 13 patients with 11 controls and showed improvement in tremor and improved function at 12 months in the treated group. Side effects are more common in bilateral procedures (often required in MS) and may occur in up to 45 percent of patients. Possible side effects include hemiparesis, dysphasia, and dysphagia in up to 10 percent of patients. Experience suggests that optimum results are obtained in patients with relatively stable disease, good mobility, and minimal overall disability status—an extremely small group.

Thalamic stimulation has been shown to alleviate tremor in up to 69 percent of patients in studies involving 13, 5, and 15 patients, respectively. Patients were carefully selected; for example, in one study the 5 patients reported were from an initial group of 17 patients, and no control study has yet been carried out. Serious side effects may occur. In one recent study comparing thalamic stimulation with lesioning, it is suggested that stimulation is associated with fewer side effects. Other approaches, including extracranial application of brief AC-pulsed electromagnetic fields, dynamic systems with multi-degree of freedom orthoses, and robotic arms based on virtual reality, have not been adequately evaluated.

In the view of the Committee, ataxia and associated tremor are among the most resistant and disabling symptoms to manage. Current strategies are of limited benefit, but information on the benefits of surgical intervention is accumulating.

Fatigue

Fatigue, which may be defined as an overwhelming sense of tiredness, lack of energy, and feelings of exhaustion in excess of what might be expected for the associated level of activity, is thought to be the most common and perhaps the most disabling symptom in MS. Fatigue must be distinguished from depression, although not infrequently these two conditions coexist and aggravate each other. Practical issues such as a poor sleep pattern resulting from painful spasms or nocturia also need to be considered. Attempts have been made to distinguish the different types of fatigue in MS, for example, that which follows activity, chronic fatigue, and fatigue associated with a clinical relapse. The underlying mechanisms remain unclear. A range of measures from generic to disease-specific are currently available to evaluate this difficult symptom, some of which are shown in Table 4-1.

Fatigue management programs are the mainstay in the management of this symptom—identifying fatigue as a relevant and disabling symptom, and examining daily routine to determine how best to minimize its impact, including energy conservation and work simplification techniques. A graded exercise program has been advocated, although there are limited data to support its usefulness. A study that evaluated the role of aerobic exercise, while showing benefit in maximum aerobic capacity and isometric muscle strength, did not show an effect on fatigue as measured by the Fatigue Impact Scale. However, two recent studies decreased fatigue, a secondary outcome, as measured by the Short Form-36 (SF-36) with exercise.

Medication for Fatigue

Three oral agents, amantadine, an antiviral agent that also has anti-parkinsonian effects, pemoline, a CNS stimulant, and modafinil, an agent effective in narcolepsy, have been studied in the management of fatigue. A small, cross-over, randomized, control trial of amantadine showed that it had a significant effect on fatigue in relation to placebo. In contrast, a small, randomized, cross-over trial of 40 patients comparing pemoline and placebo showed no significant effect from pemoline, which was poorly

Table 4-1: Levels of Measurement and Examples of Generic and MS-Specific Measures

Term	Definition	Outcome Measures	
		Generic	MS-Specific
Impairment	Clinical signs/ symptoms re- sulting from nervous sys- tem damage		Functional system of EDSS MS Functional Composite Scale (T25 FW, 9HP, PASAT)
Disability Ability	Limitations on activities of daily living from neuro- logical im- pairment	Barthel Index (BI) Functional In- dependence Measure/ Functional As- sessment Measure (FIM/FAM)	Guy's Neuro- logical Disabil- ity Scale (GNDS) MS Impair- ment Scale (MSIS)
Handicap (Participation)	Social and en- vironmental consequences from impair- ment and dis- ability	London Handi- cap Scale (LHS)	Environmental Status Scale (ESS)

Table 4-1: *(continued)*

Term	Definition	Outcome Measures Generic	MS-Specific
Health-related quality of life (QoL)	The satisfaction that people have with health-related dimensions of life, from their own perspective	Short Form-36 (SF-36) Nottingham Health Profile Sickness Impact Profile	MS Impact Scale, MS Walking Scale, MSQoL54*, Functional Assessment of MS QoL Instrument (FAMS)*, MS QoL Inventory (MSQLI)*, Functional Assessment of MS
Emotional well-being		General Health Questionnaire	
Symptoms e.g., fatigue	Overwhelming sense of tiredness or exhaustion in excess of what might be expected from level of activity	Fatigue Impact Scale Fatigue Severity Scale	MS-Specific Fatigue Scale
Spasticity	Velocity dependent increase in tonic stretch reflexes	Ashworth Scale	MS Spasticity Scale (MSSS-88)

* Developed from existing scales

tolerated in 25 percent of patients. In the most comprehensive study to date, pemoline and amantadine were compared with placebo. The placebo group received advice on fatigue management. A range of outcome measures, including the generic Fatigue Severity Scale and the six-item MS-Specific Fatigue Scale, was used.

Amantadine showed a benefit over placebo in the MS-Specific Fatigue Scale but not the Fatigue Severity Scale. No benefit was seen with pemoline. On the basis of this study, the authors suggested that amantadine should be the first-line medication for use in MS-related fatigue, although they did caution that a placebo response from either agent is a strong possibility. More recently, encouraging results have been reported from the use of modafinil. In a single-blind crossover study of 72 patients with MS, significant benefit was seen with both 200 mg and 400 mg doses with no added benefit from the higher dose and no serious side effects.

Another agent that holds some promise, although it has never been comprehensively evaluated in fatigue, is the potassium channel blocker 4-aminopyridine. This drug was comprehensively evaluated in a randomized, placebo-controlled, double-blind, cross-over study involving 70 patients with MS. A significant effect on the Expanded Disability Status Scale (EDSS) was seen in the treated group, although side effects, which included paresthesias, dizziness, and gait instability, were common. Longer follow-up has suggested that it may be useful in fatigue, although the occasional occurrence of an epileptic seizure (usually associated with high levels) remains a concern. A recent double-blind, placebo-controlled, randomized, cross-over trial involving 54 patients with progressive MS only showed an effect on the Fatigue Severity Scale in those with high serum levels of 4-AP. A number of small studies of 3-4 diaminopyridine have also suggested some potential benefit. Epileptic seizures can also result from these therapies. It has also been suggested that the disease modifying agents may improve fatigue most notably glatiramer acetate, though this remains to be proven.

A comprehensive strategy is contained within the evidence-based guidelines on fatigue management produced by the MSCCPG.

In the view of the Committee, fatigue remains one of the most disabling symptoms in MS, and drug therapy plays a relatively minor role in comparison to more practical approaches to its management.

Bladder Dysfunction

Bladder problems are among the most disabling and distressing symptoms in MS. Studies of large groups of patients have suggested that bladder dysfunction occurs in at least 70 percent of those with MS, which perhaps is not surprising given that bladder function is regulated at three interconnected levels of the CNS: the frontal lobes, the pontine micturition center, and the sacral micturition center. Bladder dysfunction in MS usually, although not invariably, results from spinal cord disease and is therefore often associated with sexual dysfunction and pyramidal symptoms such as weakness and spasticity. Urinary urgency and frequency are the most common symptoms, although hesitancy and nocturia may also be problematic. The underlying problems have been described as difficulty with storage and emptying, the former resulting from detrusor hyperreflexia and the latter from detrusor-sphincter dyssynergia.

The management of bladder dysfunction in MS includes two key components: the use of clean intermittent self-catheterization (CISC) to manage incomplete emptying, and anticholinergic agents such as oxybutynin to reduce the hyperreflexia that results in inadequate storage. However, because oxybutynin may decrease bladder emptying and therefore increase residual volume, it is important to check the residual before embarking on treatment.

CISC, which was initially introduced in the management of spinal injury, usually is taught by an experienced continence advisor but does depend on the patient's learning a consistently clean technique. Problems may arise if there is severe cognitive impairment. There are potential practical difficulties if hand function is affected by weakness or tremor, or if there is severe adductor spasticity or spasm. Some patients are unhappy about carrying out CISC, and a suprapubic vibrator is a possible alternative for those who are ambulatory. This hand-held, battery-operated device has been shown to reduce the residual volume in 80 percent of ambulant patients.

Only when adequate bladder emptying is achieved can drug treatment for detrusor hyperreflexia be initiated. The anticholinergic agent oxybutynin is the first-line treatment and has been shown to be more effective than propantheline in a small randomized trial involving 34 patients. It usually is commenced at 2.5 mg twice daily, but even this dose may cause dry mouth. The maximum recommended dose is 5 mg three times daily. A long-acting preparation that is taken once daily is available in some countries. Of the other anticholinergic drugs, tolterodine tartrate is a useful alternative to oxybutynin and is given in a dose of 2 mg twice a day or as a long-acting preparation: tolteridone LA, 4 mg daily. Occasionally, adding imipramine to oxybutynin may be helpful.

If oxybutynin is not helpful or inappropriate, desmopressin may be considered, particularly for nocturia. This synthetic antidiuretic hormone is administered by nasal spray. Several crossover studies involving relatively small numbers of patients (17 and 22, respectively) have shown that one to two puffs (10–20 µg) at bedtime or during the day can reduce urine output for 6 to 8 hours. Benefit over a prolonged period of time has been described recently in a cohort of 19 patients. The expected side effect of hyponatremia is rarely symptomatic, although headache or malaise should be taken as a warning sign. Extreme caution should be exercised in the over-65 age group, who are more likely to become symptomatic. Wheelchair-bound patients with dependent edema are also at risk of developing water retention because their nocturnal frequency may simply be an indication of resorption of edematous fluid. Desmopressin must never be taken more than once every 24 hours.

In more severe disease, interruption of the spinal pathways leads to the emergence of a new reflex at the sacral level mediated by unmyelinated C fibers that stimulates the detrusor, without the control of the normal inhibitory spinal fibers. This detrusor hyperreflexia may be reduced by the neurotoxic effects of capsaicin on the C fibers, and in a small study an instillation of 1 or 2 mmol of capsaicin dissolved in alcohol has shown a beneficial effect lasting up to five months. Repeated instillations may be required and do not appear to be responsible for any long-term side effects. Attempts have been made to evaluate the potential benefits of an ultra-potent capsinoid substance, resiniferotoxin, but these have not been successful. A pilot study of a sublingual cannabis preparation has shown some benefit in 15 patients, but this has not yet been demonstrated in more rigorous studies. Intradetrusor injection of botulinum toxin is showing considerable promise in reducing hyperactivity and the sensation of urge. However, data from randomized controlled trials are awaited.

Biofeedback has also been evaluated in a small study of 20 MS patients, which has suggested some benefit. Pelvic floor rehabilitation combined with electrostimulation was evaluated in an open, controlled, randomized study of two parallel groups with 25 women and 15 men in each group. The treatment arm underwent six sessions of electrostimulation of the pelvic floor muscles followed by regular pelvic floor exercises for 6 months. Symptoms of urinary urgency, frequency, and incontinence were significantly reduced in the treated group; this was particularly striking in the male patients.

Permanent catheterization may be necessary in many patients with severe disease as medical treatments become ineffective or impractical. A long-term urethral catheter is rarely advisable because it is likely to be extruded and destroy the bladder neck mechanism. The preferred alternative is a suprapubic catheter, which should be inserted by a urological surgeon and subsequently changed every 2 months.

In the view of the Committee, bladder symptoms usually are amenable to management; anticholinergic agents and self-catheterization are two of the most common approaches.

Bowel Dysfunction

Up to two-thirds of all people with MS complain of bowel dysfunction, frequently in combination with bladder problems. The most common symptoms are constipation and fecal incontinence, which frequently coexist. Understanding of the underlying pathophysiologic mechanisms is limited, and little if any evaluation of management strategies has taken place. Possible mechanisms resulting in constipation include slow colonic transit time, abnormal rectal function, and intussusception; incontinence may result from absent or decreased sensation of rectal filling, poor voluntary contraction of the anal sphincter–pelvic floor, or reduced rectal compliance. Factors unrelated to MS such as obstetric injury to the anal sphincters may also play a role. There are no published studies on the effect of medication on bowel symptoms in MS. Most patients try laxatives and enemas before reporting constipation. Increased dietary fiber or bulk laxatives such as lactulose may be helpful in mild constipation but are unlikely to be of benefit for severe symptoms. Stimulant or osmotic laxatives such as senna and bisacodyl may be useful. Establishing a bowel program is often advocated, although without supportive evidence.

When symptoms of fecal incontinence are mild, infrequent, and not due to impaction with overflow, treatment with loperamide or codeine phosphate may be effective, although these agents must be used with caution if incontinence coexists with constipation. An enema given in the morning may reduce the risk of incontinence during the day.

Evidence-based guidelines have recently been published by the MSCCPG and form the basis for much, although not all, of the content of this section.

In the view of the Committee, bowel dysfunction in patients with MS remains difficult to manage, with little evidence-based guidance.

Sexual Dysfunction

Sexual dysfunction is a common and very distressing symptom that affects up to 70 percent of men and women with MS. It is now discussed more openly and constructively than in the past. Some evidence to support a counseling intervention has been provided recently. There has also been an increase in the understanding of the mechanisms responsible for the symptoms and advances in treatment, although mainly in erectile dysfunction in men. Apart from specific neurological damage, the development of disability may have a major effect on the self-image of patients, which may in turn affect both their relationships and sexual function.

Management of Sexual Dysfunction in Women

The most frequently described symptoms include decreased sexual desire, diminished orgasm, difficulties with vaginal lubrication, and fatigue that interferes with sexual activity. Decreased vaginal lubrication can be treated with water-soluble lubricants, and dysesthesias may be relieved with carbamazepine or phenytoin. However, nitrergic nerves are also present in the corpus cavernosum of the clitoris and vaginal wall, so there is good rationale for expecting sildenafil (Viagra®) to have a beneficial effect. A randomized control trial is currently under way.

Management of Sexual Dysfunction in Men

Erectile difficulties are present in between 60 and 80 percent of men with MS, with symptoms ranging from difficulty sustaining an erection for intercourse, with normal nocturnal erections, to total failure of erectile function and difficulty with ejaculation in more severe disease. Clinical and neurophysiologic evidence strongly suggests a spinal origin of these symptoms. Up to 96 percent of patients have pyramidal tract signs, while physiological abnormalities implicating spinal involvement are seen in 85 percent of patients.

The value of discussing and providing relevant information cannot be underestimated.

Oral Treatments for Sexual Dysfunction

Recent advances in drug treatment, notably sildenafil (Viagra®), which has superseded all previously available therapy, are likely to have a major effect on the impact of this symptom. Release of nitric oxide from nerves supplying the arterioles of the corpora cavernosa increases intracellular levels of cyclic GMP, which results in smooth muscle relaxation and penile erection. The effect of cGMP is terminated by the enzyme phosphodiesterase, and sildenafil is an orally active inhibitor of this enzyme. A double-blind, randomized, placebo-controlled trial of 217 men with clinically definite MS with disability ranging between 2.0 and 6.0 on the EDSS has been carried out. The 16-week study included a 4-week run-in period. Patients were randomized to either placebo or 50 mg sildenafil to be taken 1 hour before intercourse at a maximum of once per day. The dose could be altered to either 100 mg or 25 mg, depending on therapeutic response and tolerability. The primary outcome measure was the International Index of Erectile Function (IIEF). One hundred and two of the 104 patients (98 percent) in the active arm completed treatment compared with 88 of the 113 patients (77 percent) receiving placebo.

The ability to achieve and maintain erections was significantly improved in the treatment group compared with controls ($p<0.0001$), and in those patients with improved erections (sildenafil responders) 92 percent reported an improvement in the ability to have satisfactory sexual activity. Adverse events were predominantly mild in nature, with headache (23.1 percent active group versus 5.3 percent in the placebo arm) and flushing (13.5

percent versus 1.8 percent) being the most common. There were three serious adverse events in each arm, none of which were thought to relate to the treatment. No cardiac symptoms were experienced in the treatment arm, although one patient in the placebo arm had a myocardial infarction during the study. A beneficial effect on related aspects of quality of life was also detected using the Life Satisfaction Checklist and the Erection Distress Scale. The treated group showed significant benefit in five of the eight components of the checklist, including life as a whole ($p<0.001$) and sexual life ($p<0.001$), but also partnership relation ($p<0.001$), family life ($p<0.003$), and social contacts ($p<0.03$).

Studies of this agent in women with sexual dysfunction suggest that sildenafil may be beneficial in a proportion of patients, particularly when lubrication is an issue.

More recently other agents with a similar mode of action but which may be more potent have become available, notably vardenafil and tadalafil. There is some evidence to suggest that vardenafil may be effective in patients who are unresponsive to sildenafil.

The only available agent that is claimed to improve ejaculatory function is yohimbine, which is thought to be an alpha-sympathetic agonist, but it has never been subjected to rigorous evaluation.

Other Approaches to the Treatment of Sexual Dysfunction

Intracorporeal pharmacotherapy has been in existence for almost two decades, initially with papaverine but more recently with prostaglandin E1 (alprostadil) at a dose of 20 µg. The latter is rapidly metabolized so that priapism and local fibrosis are very rare. Studies have shown it to be highly efficacious, with few, if any, systemic side effects. However, the disadvantages of having to inject are obvious, and patients frequently report penile pain with this treatment. There is also the option to use a medicated urethral system for erection that delivers a pellet of alprostadil into the urethra via a small applicator.

A mixture of nitric oxide–releasing dilatory creams has been evaluated in a placebo-controlled, cross-over study and was beneficial in 58 percent of men, while only 8 percent responded to the placebo. Vacuum pumps are occasionally used but have never been evaluated, and prosthetic surgery is not recommended in patients with MS.

In the view of the Committee, sexual dysfunction in men, particularly difficulty maintaining an erection, is now treated relatively easily. However, sexual dysfunction in women remains difficult to manage.

Pain

Pain is another common symptom in MS and occurs in over 50 percent of patients, with considerable impact on their quality of life. The pain is acute and usually paroxysmal in 15 percent of patients, while in the vast majority of patients it is chronic in nature. Rarely, it may be the presenting symptom. Trigeminal neuralgia is the most common type of acute pain and occurs 300 times more frequently in the MS population than in patients without MS. Lhermitte's symptom and painful tonic spasm may also be included in this category. Chronic pain consists mainly of low back pain resulting from proximal weakness and abnormal posture and gait, pain associated with spasticity, and spasm and dysesthetic extremity pain.

Carbamazepine is the mainstay of treatment of trigeminal neuralgia, whether MS-related or not. If this drug is ineffective or poorly tolerated, there is some evidence to suggest that other anticonvulsants may be useful, particularly phenytoin. Small studies of misoprostol, a prostaglandin E1 analogue, have suggested partial benefit in patients who respond poorly to carbamazepine. Gabapentin and lamotrigine also have been reported to be of some benefit. Pain becomes chronic in a small proportion of patients, and surgical intervention may be required in this group, particularly if drug therapy is less than adequate or poorly tolerated. Percutaneous procedures have shown benefit, although reinjection may be necessary. This approach has not been rigorously evaluated. Logically, microvascular decompression should not have a role, although recent studies have suggested benefit in about 50 percent of those selected for treatment. Chronic pain is more difficult to treat, although there is some evidence to support the use of amitriptyline in dysesthetic pain, followed by carbamazepine, clonazepam, and other anticonvulsant drugs. Physiotherapy to improve proximal stability and incorporate education on improved posture in standing and sitting is the cornerstone of treatment for low back pain. Nonsteroidal anti-inflammatory drugs, transcutaneous electrical nerve stimulation (TENS), and a heating pad may all play a useful subsidiary role. A recent pilot study of the oral synthetic delta-9-tetrahydrocannabinol dronabinol suggested some benefit in central pain in MS.

In the view of the Committee, acute paroxysmal pain usually responds to carbamazepine, and other drugs are also available. Chronic pain is more difficult to manage and is often undertreated. It frequently requires multidisciplinary input and, if severe, may benefit from the expertise of a pain clinic.

Other Paroxysmal Symptoms

Although relatively uncommon, other paroxysmal symptoms are highly characteristic of MS and include paroxysmal dysarthria and ataxia, tonic spasms, and paroxysmal sensory symptoms. These symptoms are thought to relate to ephaptic transmission; they last less than 2 minutes but may occur frequently (sometimes up to 20 to 30 times a day) for a 2- to 6-week period. They are exquisitely sensitive to carbamazepine, and a small study has suggested that gabapentin may be a useful alternative. Bromocriptine also has been mentioned in case reports.

Epilepsy occurs in about 5 percent of people with MS, and although this may be coincidental in some cases, there is evidence to suggest that it relates to either cortical or subcortical lesions or very large plaques that behave like space-occupying lesions and usually occur in advanced disease. Treatment should be with anticonvulsants, although their use need not always be prolonged, particularly if there is only a short cluster of attacks in association with an acute inflammatory lesion that subsequently resolves.

Cognitive Symptoms

Cognitive deficits occur in up to 60 percent of people with MS and affect attention, conceptual reasoning, executive function, visuospatial perception, and recent memory, with relative sparing of language and intellectual function. They have a major impact on all aspects of functioning, particularly employment, and, if severe, may limit the benefits of rehabilitation. Assessment and identification of particular deficits are fundamental to developing strategies to overcome or compensate for them. A cognitive rehabilitation program in which communication skills training included a combination of cognitive rehabilitation and cognitive-behavioral psychotherapy has been described but not yet evaluated. There is little evidence available on the treatment of specific cognitive deficits. The effects of cognitive training and psychotherapy have been evaluated in a small randomized study of 40 patients, but no clear benefit could be determined apart from an apparent improvement in mood in the treatment arm. A computer-based retraining program has been reported to have some short-term benefit (9 weeks) in specific attention deficits and related activities of daily living in a study of 22 patients. A recent randomized, double-blind, placebo-controlled trial of computer-aided retraining of memory and attention involving 82 patients did not show benefit. The only medication to be studied in this regard is 4-aminopyridine, but no significant benefit was seen in a small randomized, double-blind, placebo-controlled, cross-over study of 20 patients.

A small exploratory study looked at the potential for the acetyl cholinesterase inhibitor rivastigmine to encourage plasticity in patients with cognitive impairment and suggested that it might help the brain to adapt. Further research is needed to follow this up. Recently another agent, donepezil, has been studied in a single-center, double-blind, placebo-controlled trial involving 69 patients with MS. Patients received 10 mg donepezil for 24 weeks or placebo and were evaluated across a range of cognitive tests that addressed verbal learning, memory, word fluency, spatial recall, and executive function. Affect and fatigue were also measured. A moderate treatment effect was seen in memory performance but not in any of the other domains. Patients also felt they had improved although there was an element of un-blinding.

In the view of the Committee, these are particularly important symptoms, and it is encouraging to see that they are now recognized as such. More active approaches to management are urgently needed, including larger trials of drug treatments.

Psychiatric and Psychological Dysfunction

Psychiatric morbidity is increased in MS, with over 50 percent of patients being symptomatic at some stage. Irritability, poor concentration, depressed mood, and anxiety are the most common symptoms. The depressive symptoms may not be severe, and only a minority of patients requires medication. The treatment of depression is similar to that for people who do not have MS, and there are few randomized controlled trials of antidepressants in MS. A study of desipramine showed moderate efficacy, but the dose was limited by anticholinergic side effects.

Psychological disturbances are common in MS, and many patients have difficulty coping from the time of initial diagnosis. This may be compounded by the subsequent development of disability. Different methods for treating psychological difficulties have been described, but few have been evaluated. The role of psychotherapy in MS has been described, and the role of group psychotherapy has been evaluated in a small group of patients with MS. Some benefit was seen in relation to "locus of control," but no effect was seen in anxiety or self-esteem. A number of small studies have suggested that exercise may improve symptoms such as depression, anxiety, and anger.

In the view of the Committee, these symptoms need to be actively identified and managed, although this may not involve drug treatment.

Other Symptoms

Visual Dysfunction

Although optic neuritis, the most common visual symptom, usually is transient and associated with good recovery, some patients have persisting and occasionally progressive deficits and may benefit from referral to a low vision clinic. Involuntary eye movement disorders, such as nystagmus and oscillopsia, also cause distressing visual disturbance. These symptoms may be helped by the use of prisms, and there is anecdotal evidence to suggest the use of a number of medications including baclofen, gabapentin, and isoniazid. A small study has evaluated the role of the glutamate agonist memantine in pendular nystagmus, and all 11 patients treated with this agent were reported as showing a positive response.

Vertigo

Dizziness or vertigo may occur as part of a brain stem relapse and may be accompanied by nystagmus and ataxia, resulting in a profound reduction in mobility and safety. Prochlorperazine may be helpful in acute vertigo, while physiotherapy, including Cawthorne-Cooksey exercises, together with cinnarizine, may be helpful when symptoms are chronic.

Swallowing, Speech, and Respiratory Dysfunction

Dysphagia is not uncommon in MS, and suggestive symptoms have been reported in up to 43 percent of the MS population. These symptoms included coughing when eating, choking, anxiety about swallowing, and change in swallowing function. Such symptoms are often overlooked until the patient has a severe choking episode. Mild dysphagia usually is easily managed with assessment and advice from a speech therapist. There is an unquantified risk of aspiration pneumonia in more severe cases, and investigation may include videofluoroscopy. Percutaneous gastrostomy may be required if swallowing is unsafe or intake is inadequate.

Speech disturbance in MS usually is due to dysarthria, although dysphasia does occasionally occur, usually in patients with severe cognitive deficits. Again, assessment and management by a speech therapist is helpful, and a communication aid may be useful in very severe dysarthria.

Respiratory insufficiency may occur in advanced MS but also may complicate acute brain stem episodes. Respiratory muscle weakness, including diaphragmatic weakness, is the most common cause. Respiratory support may be required in an acute event, while in more chronic situations the patient may be taught to incorporate the diaphragm when talking.

Temperature Sensitivity

Many patients report a worsening of symptoms associated with an increase in temperature or exercise, particularly in relation to visual function (Uhthoff's phenomenon). The drug 4-aminopyridine has been reported to be particularly beneficial in patients with temperature sensitivity. Practical advice about air-conditioning systems may be helpful, and the use of a cooling suit might be considered if the symptoms are very severe (see Chapter 5). A recent randomized, double-blind, controlled study of cooling therapy has been reported. It included 84 patients with mild to moderate disability, together with heat sensitivity, and looked at the benefit of a single dose of cooling therapy and at more sustained therapy over a month. Some benefits were seen in mobility and visual testing in both the acute and sustained treatment, and benefit in fatigue was reported in the latter group.

NEUROREHABILITATION

The preceding section underlines the wide range of symptoms that may occur in MS, many of which coexist and interact. A successful management strategy must account for the complex pattern of disability that results, together with the possibility that treating one symptom may worsen another. It also is apparent that comprehensive management will invariably require a number of different approaches, including the provision of information, patient education, therapy from a range of disciplines, and drug treatment. Finally, the variable and fluctuating nature of MS means that the needs of the individual patient will change over time, often quite abruptly, and, for many, these needs will increase over time.

   The philosophy of rehabilitation, which emphasizes patient education and self-management, is ideally suited to meet the complex and variable needs of MS. Rehabilitation aims to improve independence and quality of life by maximizing ability and participation. It has been defined by the World Health Organization as "an active process by which those disabled by injury or disease achieve a full recovery or if a full recovery is not possible realize their optimal physical, mental and social potential and are integrated into their most appropriate environment."

   The essential components of successful rehabilitation include:

1.   Expert multidisciplinary assessment

2.   Goal-orientated programs

3.   Evaluation of impact on patient and goal achievement

The philosophy of rehabilitation applies at every stage of the condition, from initial diagnosis to the management of those with severe disability. In order to provide a framework to consider the needs of people with MS, it is helpful to divide the condition into four stages:

1. Diagnosis

2. Minimal disability

3. Moderate disability

4. Severe disability

There are consistent themes running through each of these stages, including:

- Access to up-to-date information

- Appropriate expertise – often of a multidisciplinary nature

- Flexibility and accessibility

- Good communication

- Empowering the person with MS

Measuring Outcome

Evaluating the outcome from interventions at any stage of MS is extremely challenging but also of the greatest importance if there is to be ongoing improvement in the process and impact of rehabilitation. Evaluating the effect on the patient requires the use of outcome measures that are scientifically sound (reliable, valid, and responsive) and clinically useful (short, simple, etc.). They also must be appropriate to the sample under study and the intervention being evaluated. In the case of neurorehabilitation, the potential effects are not expected at the levels of pathology and impairment but rather in improving activity and participation (WHO ICIDH 2) and in enhancing the broader, more patient-oriented areas of quality of life, coping skills, and self-efficacy. It is particularly important that the perspective of the patient is incorporated into the measure in a scientifically sound manner.

The standard outcome measure in therapeutic trials in MS, Kurtzke's EDSS is inappropriate for evaluating rehabilitation not only because of its scientific limitations (particularly poor responsiveness) but also because it does not measure many of the relevant areas, such as fatigue and cognition, and does not incorporate the perspective of the patient. Consequently, a number of generic measures of disability/ability (Barthel Index [BI], Functional Independence Measure [FIM], Functional Independence Measure/Functional Assessment Measure [FIM/FAM]), participation/handicap (London Handicap Scale [LHS]), and health-related quality of life (The Short Form 36 Health Survey Questionnaire [SF-36]) have been used in MS rehabilitation (Table 4-1).

More recently, a number of MS-specific measures have been developed that are currently undergoing evaluation. These address disability (UK Disability Scale; MS Functional Composite – PASAT, 9 hole peg test and 10 metre times walk; MS Walking Scale), health related quality of life (MS Quality of Life Inventory, Functional Assessment of MS [FAMS], MS QOL 54, The Leeds QOL Scale, the MS Disease Impact Scale (MSIS).

These scales do not, however, capture the area of goal achievement, an essential component of the rehabilitation process. This may be done through using integrated care pathways (ICPs). An ICP is an excellent audit tool that documents when goals are not achieved on time but more usefully indicates why this has occurred, such as the underestimation of cognitive dysfunction or the impact of fatigue.

Diagnostic Phase

This is known to be a time of great anxiety and concern, and until recently was particularly badly managed. There are now accepted standards laid out in a number of recent documents. These are quite logical and include:

- Certain, clear diagnosis
- Appropriate support at diagnosis
- Access to information
- Continuing education

New diagnostic criteria have recently been developed that incorporate more fully the evidence from MRI and allow an earlier diagnosis. The process by which the diagnosis is made and communicated to the patient has been greatly enhanced by the introduction of MS nurse specialists and the establishment of diagnostic clinics, which are lead by neurologists with an interest in MS and allow relevant investigations, including MRI to be carried out on the same day. This service also incorporates links with the MS Society, the provision of written information, a telephone help-line, and continuing support and education in the form of regular classes. This model ensures that standards are met and proves to be both efficient and cost-effective.

Conclusion: The time of diagnosis is a crucial stage for people with MS. Recent improvements in the diagnostic criteria and the way in which this critical time is managed are particularly welcome.

Minimal Disability

Following diagnosis many patients will have a period of a decade or more when they have regular relapses but little or no disability. They will have a number of needs during this time, which include access to:

- Advice, support, and information
- Self-management options
- Treatment of relapses including disease-modifying agents
- Treatment of other conditions

The main focus should be on self-management, with an emphasis on the concept of wellness incorporating diet, exercise, and a healthy lifestyle. A number of studies have been carried out evaluating the role of aerobic exercise, resistive exercise, and more recently a training program. The impact of aerobic exercise was evaluated in 46 patients with relatively mild MS. Twenty-one patients were randomly assigned to a 15-week exercise program, while 25 patients had no exercise during that period. There was a wide range of outcome measures, including aerobic capacity, isometric strength, a quality-of-life measure, the Sickness Impact Profile (SIP), the Fatigue Severity Scales (FSS), and the EDSS. Significant changes from baseline were seen in the exercise group over the 15 weeks in the physiologic measures and the physical component of the SIP. There was little sustained change in the psychosocial domain of the SIP and none in the EDSS or FSS.

Recently, the effects of a short-term exercise program on aerobic fitness, fatigue, and health perception was evaluated in a group of 26 patients and the results compared to 26 matched healthy controls. Although compliance was low (65 percent), benefits were seen in all areas and the regime did not result in symptom exacerbation. Significant benefit was seen in two domains of the SF-36: vitality and social functioning.

Few studies have looked at therapy intervention in the management of MS, and the only specific modality examined has been physiotherapy. A randomized control trial of inpatient physiotherapy (6.5 hours over 2 weeks) was carried out on 45 patients. Outcome measures included the Rivermead Mobility Index, the Barthel ADL Index, and a visual analogue scale (VAS) of "mobility-related distress." The only measure to demonstrate a significant benefit in the treated group was the VAS. A second study went a step further and attempted to compare two forms of physiotherapy. This pilot study involved 23 patients, 20 of whom completed the study. Ten patients received what was described as an impairment-based "facilitation approach" (e.g., Bobath), while the other group had a more disability-based task-orientated approach (e.g., Carr and Shepherd). Patients received a minimum of 15 sessions over 5 to 7 weeks. The outcome measures were mobility-based and included the 10-meter timed walk and the Rivermead Mobility Index. Not surprisingly, no difference was seen between the two small groups, but both improved from baseline ($p<0.05$).

A recent randomized, controlled, cross-over study evaluated hospital and home-based physiotherapy in 40 MS patients with mobility problems. A very wide range of outcome measures was used, but physiotherapy resulted in significant benefit, irrespective of location, on the Rivermead Mobility Index, which was supported by other measures of mobility, gait, and balance. There was no difference between treatment at home (the patient's preference) or in the hospital, although the latter was less expensive.

Finally in this group of minimally affected patients it is important to remember that although the majority of relapses resolve completely, up to 40 percent may leave some residual problems. Therefore while steroids might hasten the role of recovery from a relapse, there is a role for therapy input and possibly involvement of the multidisciplinary team in those with residual deficit. A recent randomized, controlled trial has shown that in patients who have not recovered fully following a relapse, there is a significant benefit from therapy input in addition to steroids when compared to steroids alone. Audit data from a neurorehabilitation service also supports the role of rehabilitation in those who have developed severe disability following a relapse.

Conclusion: There is increasing evidence to support the role of a range of therapy inputs at this stage of MS, but larger and more rigorous studies need to be carried out.

Moderate Disability

This population of patients has the greater needs in the management of its increasing disability. These include:

- Rehabilitation and symptomatic management
- Easy access to responsive and coordinated services

- Appropriate level of expertise
- Good communication
- Self-management

A comprehensive rehabilitation program may be particularly appropriate although its evaluation may prove challenging. The difficulties of evaluating any intervention within the context of a randomized, double-blind, placebo-controlled trial in a variable and unpredictable condition such as MS were outlined in Chapter 1. Evaluating as broad an area as neurorehabilitation, which at the same time has to meet the specific needs of an individual patient, poses additional problems in trial design. Chief among these are a lack of detailed description (e.g., number of disciplines involved, techniques employed, etc.) and inadequate standardization of input, including its duration and location (inpatient, outpatient, or community-based). There also is reluctance among therapists to use a control group, and limited resources often prohibit the use of independent assessors, which is particularly important when blinding is so difficult and perhaps even impossible. Finally, there is no consensus as to the most appropriate outcome measures, and until recently there has been inconsistent use of limited and often inappropriate tools.

Despite these obstacles, it is possible to attempt some degree of evaluation, as has been demonstrated by a number of recent studies, although many more are required.

The two key questions that need to be answered are:

1. Is comprehensive rehabilitation effective in improving ability, participation, and quality of life?

2. If so, do these benefits carry over in the medium to long term?

The majority of studies have evaluated inpatient rehabilitation, which may be more accessible for study design. Of the nine studies of in-patient rehabilitation listed in Table 4-2, three are of single group design, although all suggest potential benefit from rehabilitation in the area of disability.

Table 4-2: Summary of Recent Outcome Studies of Comprehensive Rehabilitation in People with MS

Study	Study Design	Sample	Main Outcomes/ Instruments	Time of Assessments	Results
Inpatient Rehabilitation					
Franca-bandera et al.	Prospective, stratified, randomized study	84	ISS. Need for home assistance (hours)	Admission and at 3-month intervals for 2 years	Preliminary results suggest marginal benefit in inpatient group
Kidd et al.	Prospective, single-group, pre-and post-study design	79	DSS, Barthel Index, ESS	Admission and discharge	Significant improvement in disability and handicap
Freeman et al.	Prospective, single group, longitudinal study design	50 (prog MS)	EDSS and FS, FIM, LHS, SF-36, GHQ-28	Admission and discharge and at 3-month intervals for 1 year	Benefits in disability, handicap, QoL and emotional well-being persist for 6–9 months

(continued)

Table 4-2: *(continued)*

Study	Study Design	Sample	Main Outcomes/ Instruments	Time of Assessments	Results
Solari et al.	Randomized single group study comparing inpatient and home exercise programme	50 (ambulatory)	EDSS, FIM, SF-36	Baseline, 3, 9 and 15 weeks	Benefits in disability and some aspects of QoL
Aisen et al.	Retrospective, single group, pre- and post- study design	37	EDSS and FS, FIM	Admission, discharge and telephone follow-up (between 6 and 36 months post discharge)	Significant improvement in both FIM and EDSS
Kidd, Thompson	Prospective, single- group, pre- and post- study design	47	EDSS, FIM, ESS	Admission, discharge and 3- month follow-up	Gains in disability maintained at 3 months; Handicap improved over study period

Table 4-2: *(continued)*

Study	Study Design	Sample	Main Outcomes/Instruments	Time of Assessments	Results
Freeman et al.	Stratified, randomized, wait list controlled study design	66 (prog. MS)	EDSS and FS, FIM, LHS	Baseline and 6 weeks	Significant benefit in disability and handicap
Romberg et al.	Randomized controlled study	95	Timed walk test upper and lower limb strength balance	Baseline and 6 months	Improvement in TWT and upper limb endurance
Storr et al.	Randomized, parallel group, blinded trial	90	MSIS, EDSS, GNDS, 9HP, TWT	Baseline and 10 weeks	No benefit

Outpatient Rehabilitation

Study	Study Design	Sample	Main Outcomes/Instruments	Time of Assessments	Results
Di Fabio et al.	Non-equivalent pre-test, post-test control group design	45 (prog. MS)	MS-related symptom. RIC-FAS Fatigue frequency	At entry and at 1 year	33 patients completed 1 year. Significant benefit seen in MS-related symptoms, inc fatigue

(continued)

Table 4-2: *(continued)*

Study	Study Design	Sample	Main Outcomes/ Instruments	Time of Assessments	Results
Patti et al.	Randomized, controlled trial	111	EDSS and FS, FIM, SF-36	Baseline and six weeks	Significant improvement in FIM

BUSTOP: Burke Stroke Time-oriented Profile; CRDS: Computerized Rehabilitation and Data System; DSS: Disability Status Scale; EDSS: Expanded Disability Status Scale; ESS: Environmental Status Scale; FIM: Functional Independence Measure; LORS-II: Revised Level of Rehabilitation Scale; FS: Functional Systems; ISS: Incapacity Status Scale; LHS: London Handicap Scale; SF-36: Short Form 36 Health Survey Questionnaire; GHQ-28: 28-item General Health Questionnaire; RIC-FAS: Rehabilitation Institute of Chicago Functional Assessment Scale.

The study by Freeman and co-workers was a randomized, wait-list controlled study of 66 patients with progressive MS. Patients were stratified on entry according to EDSS score, and the treatment group received a short period of inpatient rehabilitation (mean, 20 days). Measures of disability, the Functional Independence Measure (FIM), and handicap, the London Handicap Scale (LHS), were applied on entry into the study and 6 weeks later. The two groups were well matched in relation to age, sex, disease pattern, and duration, and the treated group showed a significant benefit in both disability ($p<0.001$) and handicap ($p<0.01$) when compared with the control group. No change in the EDSS score was seen in either group.

A randomized, single-blind trial compared a 3-week inpatient rehabilitation program with a home exercise program in 50 less disabled patients who were still ambulatory. Patients were evaluated with the EDSS, FIM, and SF-36, a quality-of-life measure, at baseline, 3, 6, 9, and 15 weeks. Significant benefit in disability and some aspects of quality of life (mental not physical) was seen at the end of the 3-week period in the rehabilitation group compared with those doing a home exercise program. This beneficial difference between groups was seen again at 9 weeks but had disappeared by 15 weeks.

A more recent study assessed the role of strength and aerobic training, initially as an in-patient for three weeks but followed by 23 weeks at home in patients with MS of mild to moderate severity. Benefits in mobility and upper limb endurance were seen in the intervention group when compared to controls. In contrast a study of in-patient rehabilitation showed no benefit in patients whose MS was stable.

Few researchers have attempted to evaluate outpatient-based rehabilitation in MS. One study randomly assigned 46 patients with progressive MS to an active treatment group (20 patients receiving 5 hours of outpatient therapy a week for 1 year) and to a wait-list control group. The range of outcomes used included an MS-related symptoms checklist composite score, a measure of fatigue frequency, and items from the Rehabilitation Institute of Chicago's Functional Assessment Scale. A significant reduction in the frequency of MS symptoms and fatigue was seen. A more recent randomized controlled trial of outpatient rehabilitation involved 111 patients with progressive MS. Those in the treatment arm underwent a 6-week period of treatment. The primary outcome measure was the FIM and moderately significant benefits (effect size greater than 0.4) were seen in the total score and in the sphincter, self-care, transfers, and locomotion sub-scores.

Do Benefits of Rehabilitation Carry Over in Medium Term?

Three studies have attempted to address this question and all were restricted to the evaluation of a single group. The first was a retrospective study based on reviewing inpatient records and making subsequent phone contact with 37 patients 6 to 36 months later. It suggested that gains on the EDSS and FIM documented on discharge were maintained at follow-up. The second study was a prospective evaluation of 47 patients seen 3 months post-discharge and included a measure of handicap (Environmental Status Scale) along with the EDSS and FIM. No change was seen in the EDSS during or following rehabilitation; gains in the FIM were maintained, while the level of handicap actually improved over the 3-month follow-up period.

The most recent study involved the prospective longitudinal evaluation of 50 of the patients with progressive MS involved in the randomized control trial described earlier. This study used a wider range of outcome measures; in addition to the EDSS and FIM, there were measures of handicap (LHS), quality of life (SF-36), and emotional well-being (General Health Questionnaire GHQ). Patients were evaluated for 12 months at 3-month intervals following discharge, and 12-month data were collected on 48 of the 50 patients (92 percent). As might be expected, there was great variation between individual patients as well as considerable differences between the outcome measures. Summary measures were used to calculate the time taken to return to baseline. The EDSS deteriorated from a median of 6.8 on discharge to 8.0 at 12-month follow-up. Despite this, the gains in disability were maintained for 6 months before slowly declining. As in the previous study, handicap improved further following discharge, but the benefit lessened after 6 months. Quality of life and emotional well-being improved considerably during the rehabilitation period, and this improvement was maintained for 10 and 7 months, respectively, before beginning to return to the baseline. A further finding of this study was that those who made the most gains during the rehabilitation period tended to maintain those gains for a longer time.

A final question is whether we can predict those who have the potential to benefit from neurorehabilitation or perhaps, more importantly, those who will not make gains. Two studies have addressed this issue. Both agree that severe cognitive impairment is a particular challenge and one found that severe ataxia was also associated with a poor response.

Conclusion: Although it is difficult to combine the results of all of these studies and there are major methodological differences between them, with few, if any, reaching an adequate scientific level, they all suggest that organized patient-centered multidisciplinary rehabilitation is of benefit in MS management. There is also some evidence to suggest that the gains derived from rehabilitation are maintained in the short term, at least in part, in this progressive condition. They emphasize the need for a range of outcome measures to be used and stress the importance of continuity of care.

Severe Disability

There have been few, if any, studies evaluating input in those with severe disability. Their needs include:

- Access to information and expertise

- Good communication and coordinated care

- Adequate community care services

- Flexible provision of respite care

- Appropriate long-term care facilities including palliative care

There has been recent interest in the evaluation of palliative care, which has a major role to play at this stage of the condition. There is an urgent need for more evaluation and development of services for people with severe disability.

SERVICE DELIVERY

Evaluating Service Delivery: Developing Models of Care in MS

Evaluating service delivery may be considered the most important and relevant issue in the management of MS because it incorporates acute hospital and neurorehabilitation services together with community-based activities and, in essence, has to bring together medical and social services in a way that meets the complex and ever-changing needs of the person with MS. Ideally, most services should be community-based with supporting expertise from the acute hospital or rehabilitation center at times of particular need (e.g., at diagnosis or at the time of a severe relapse) or complexity (when multiple symptoms interact and intensive inpatient rehabilitation is required). The optimum method of service delivery has not yet been defined, and little work has been done comparing existing services.

A recently published study carried out in Rome compared two forms of service delivery in a randomized controlled trial of 201 patients with MS. One group (133 patients) received what was described as "hospital" home care, in which patients remained in the community but had immediate access to the hospital-based, multidisciplinary team as and when required, while the other group (68 patients) received routine care. The range of outcomes, which included EDSS, FIM, SF-36, and measures of anxiety and mood, were carried out at baseline and at 12 months. No difference was seen in the level of disability between the two groups, but the more intensively treated patients had significantly less depression and improved quality of life.

There continue to be major problems worldwide in delivering a model of care that provides truly coordinated services. There is serious inequity of service provision both within and across countries, and an inordinate and unacceptable reliance on family and friends to provide essential care. Establishing guidance such as has been done by NICE is a step forward but a global initiative such as the MSIF principles may be more effective globally. The key challenge will be ensuring the translation of these documents into practice.

Conclusion: Although there is good empirical evidence to support coordinated expert service delivery, there is little evidence currently available to support this concept in the management of MS and further studies are required.

Guide to Further Reading

Symptomatic Management

General Reviews

- Brichetto G, Uccelli MM, Mancardi GL, Solaro C. Symptomatic medication use in multiple sclerosis. *Multiple Sclerosis* 2003; 9:458–460.

- National Institute for Clinical Excellence. Multiple Sclerosis: Management of multiple sclerosis in primary and secondary care. Clinical Guideline 8. 2003.

- Schapiro RT. *Managing the Symptoms of Multiple Sclerosis*. New York: Demos Medical Publishing, 20

- Thompson AJ. Symptomatic management and rehabilitation in multiple sclerosis. *J Neurol Neurosurg Psychiatry* 2001; 71(Suppl II):ii22–ii27.

- Thompson AJ. Neurorehabilitation in multiple sclerosis: foundations, facts and fiction. *Curr Opin Neurol* 2005; 18: 267–271.

Spasticity

- Beard S, Hunn A, Wight J. Treatments for spasticity and pain in multiple sclerosis: a systematic review. *Health Technol Assess*. 2003; 7(40): iii, ix–x, 1–111.

- Hymen N, Barnes B, Bhakta B, et al. Botulinum toxin treatment of hip adductor spasticity in multiple sclerosis: A prospective, randomized, double blind, placebo controlled dose ranging study. *J Neurol Neurosurg Psychiatry* 2000; 68:707–712.

- Jarrett L, Nandi P, Thompson AJ. Managing severe lower limb spasticity in multiple sclerosis: does intrathecal phenol have a role? *J Neurol, Neurosurg and Psychiatry* 2002; 73:705–709.

- Killestein J, Hoogervorst ELJ, Reif M, et al. Safety, tolerability and efficacy of orally administered cannabinoids in MS. *Neurology* 2002; 58:1404–1407.

- Multiple Sclerosis Council for Clinical Practice Guidelines. *Spasticity Management in Multiple Sclerosis.* Published by Consortium of MS Centres. 2003.

- Ochs G, Struppler A, Meyerson BA, et al. Intrathecal baclofen for long-term treatment of spasticity: A multicentre study. *J Neurol Neurosurg Psychiatry* 1989; 52: 933–939.

- Paisley S, Beard S, Hunn A, Wight J. Clinical effectiveness of oral treatments for spasticity in multiple sclerosis. *Multiple Sclerosis* 2002; 8:319–329.

- Penn RD, Savoy SM, Corcos D, et al. Intrathecal baclofen for severe spinal spasticity. *N Engl J Med* 1989; 320: 1517–1521.

- Salame K, Ouaknine GE, Rochkind S, Constantini S, Razon N. Surgical treatment of spasticity by selective posterior rhizotomy: 30 years experience. *Isr Med Assoc J* 2003; 5:543–546.

- Shakespeare DT, Boggild M, Young C. Anti-spasticity agents for multiple sclerosis. *Cochrane Database Syst Rev* 2003; (4):CD001332.

- Sheean G. Pathophysiology of spasticity. In: Sheean G (ed.). *Spasticity Rehabilitation.* Edinburgh: Churchill Communications Europe Ltd., 1998:17–38.

- Thompson AJ, Jarrett L, Lockley L, Marsden J, Stevenson V. Clinical management of spasticity. *J Neurol Neurosurg Psychiatry* 2005; 76:459–463.

- Vaney C, Heinzel-Gutenbrunner M, Jobin P, Tschopp F, Gattlen B, Hagen U, Schnelle M, Reif M. Efficacy, safety and tolerability of an orally administered cannabis extract in the treatment of spasticity in patients with multiple sclerosis: A randomized, double-blind, placebo-controlled, crossover study. *Multiple Sclerosis* 2004; 10: 417–424.

• Wagstaff AJ, Bryson HM. Tizanidine: A review of its pharmacology, clinical efficacy and tolerability in the management of spasticity associated with cerebral and spinal disorders. *Drugs* 1997; 53(3):435–452.

• Zajicek J, Fox P, Sanders H, Wright D, Vickery J, Nunn A, Thompson A, UK MS Research Group. Cannabinoids for treatment of spasticity and other symptoms related to multiple sclerosis (CAMS study): Multicentre randomized placebo-controlled trial. *Lancet* 2003; 362:1517–26.

• Zajicek J, Sanders HP, Wright DE, et al. Cannabinoids in multiple sclerosis (CAMS) study: safety and efficacy data for 12 months follow-up. *J Neurol Neurosurg and Psychiatry* (in press).

Ataxia

• Alusi SH, Glickman S, Aziz TZ, Bain PG. Tremor in multiple sclerosis. (Editorial) *J Neurol Neurosurg Psychiatry* 1999; 66:131–134.

• Alusi SH, Aziz TZ, Glickman S, Jahanshahi M, Stein JF, Bain PG. Stereotactic lesional surgery for the treatment of tremor in multiple sclerosis: A prospective case-controlled study. *Brain* 2001; 124:1576–1589.

• Fox P, Bain PG, Glickman S, Carroll C, Zajicek J. The effects of cannabis on tremor in patients with multiple sclerosis. *Neurology* 2004; 62:1105–1109.

• Montgomery EB, Baker KB, Kinkel RP, Barnett G. Chronic thalamic stimulation for the tremor of multiple sclerosis. *Neurology* 1999; 53:625–628.

• Rice GPA, Lescaux J, Ebers G. Ondansetron versus placebo for disabling cerebellar tremor: Final report of a randomized clinical trial. *Ann Neurol* 1999; 46:493.

- Schuurman PR, Andries Bosch D, Dossuyt PMM, et al. A comparison of continuous thalamic stimulation and thalamotomy for suppression of severe tremor. *N. Engl J Med* 2000; 343:461–468.

- Wishart HA, Roberts DW, Roth RM et al. Chronic deep brain stimulation for the treatment of tremor in multiple sclerosis: Review and case reports. *J Neurol Neurosurg and Psychiatry* 2003; 74:1392–1397.

Fatigue

- Bakshi R. Fatigue associated with multiple sclerosis: Diagnosis, impact and management. *Multiple Sclerosis* 2003; 9:219–227.

- Comi G, Leocani L, Rossi P, Colombo B. Physiopathology and treatment of fatigue in multiple sclerosis. *J Neurol* 2001; 248:174–179.

- Gillson G, Richard TL, Smith RB, Wright JV. A double-blind pilot study of the effect of Prokarin on fatigue in multiple sclerosis. *Multiple Sclerosis* 2002; 8:30–35.

- Krupp LB, Coyle PK, Doscher C, et al. Fatigue therapy in multiple sclerosis: Results of a double-blind, randomized, parallel trial of amantadine, pemoline, and placebo. *Neurology* 1995; 45(11):1956–1961.

- Krupp LB. Mechanisms, measurement, and management of fatigue in multiple sclerosis. In: Thompson AJ, Polman C, Hohlfeld R (eds.). *Multiple Sclerosis: Clinical Challenges and Controversies.* London: Martin Dunitz, 1997; 283–294.

- Metz LM, Patten SB, Archibald CJ, et al. The effect of immunomodulatory treatment on multiple sclerosis fatigue. *J Neurol Neurosurg and Psychiatry* 2004; 75:1045–1047.

- Multiple Sclerosis Council for Clinical Practice Guidelines. *Fatigue and Multiple Sclerosis.* Washington, DC: Paralyzed Veterans of America, 1998.

- Rammohan KW, Rosenberg JH, Lynn DJ, Blumenfeld AM, Pollak CP, Nagaraja HN. Efficacy and safety of modafinil (Provigil) for the treatment of fatigue in multiple sclerosis: a two centre phase 2 study. *J Neurol Neurosurg Psychiatry* 2002; 72:179–183.

- van Diemen HA, Polman CH, van Dongen TM, et al. The effect of 4-aminopyridine on clinical signs in multiple sclerosis: A randomized, placebo-controlled, double-blind, cross-over study. *Ann Neurol* 1992; 32(2): 123–130.

Bladder, Bowel and Sexual Dysfunction

- Dasgupta R, Fowler CJ. Bladder, bowel and sexual dysfunction in multiple sclerosis: management strategies *Drugs* 2003; 63:153–166.

Bladder Dysfunction

- Betts CD, D'Mellow MT, Fowler CJ. Urinary symptoms and the neurological features of bladder dysfunction in multiple sclerosis. *J Neurol Neurosurg Psychiatry* 1993; 56(3):245–250.

- Brady CM, Dasguta R, Dalton C, Wiseman OJ, Berkley KJ, Fowler CJ. An open-label pilot study of cannabis-based extracts for bladder dysfunction in advanced multiple sclerosis. *Multiple Sclerosis* 2004; 10:425–433.

- Fowler CJ. Investigation of the neurogenic bladder. *J Neurol Neurosurg Psychiatry* 1996; 60:6–13.

- Harper M, Fowler CJ, Dasgupta P. Botulinum toxin and its applications in the lower urinary tract. *BJU Int.* 2004; 93:702–704.

- MS Council for Clinical Practice Guidelines. Urinary *Dysfunction and Multiple Sclerosis. Evidence-Based Management Strategies for Urinary Dysfunction in Multiple Sclerosis.* Washington, DC: Paralyzed Veterans of America, 1998.

- Valiquette G, Herbert J, Maede D. Desmopressin in the management of nocturia in patients with multiple sclerosis. A double-blind, crossover trial. *Arch Neurol* 1996; 53:1270–1275.

- Vahtera T, Haaranen M, Viramo-Koskela AL, Ruutiainen J. Pelvic floor rehabilitation is effective in patients with multiple sclerosis. *Clin Rehabil* 1997; 11:211–219.

Bowel Dysfunction

- Fowler CJ, Henry MM. Gastrointestinal dysfunction in MS. *Semin Neurol* 1996; 16:277–279.

- Hinds JP, Eidelman BH, Wald A. Prevalence of bowel dysfunction in MS. *Gastroenterology* 1990; 98:1538–1542.

Sexual Dysfunction

- Betts CD, Jones SJ, Fowler CG, Fowler CJ. Erectile dysfunction in multiple sclerosis: Associated neurological and neurophysiological deficits, and treatment of the condition. *Brain* 1994; 117:1303–1310.

- Carson C, Hatzichristou D, Carrier S, et al. Erectile response with vardenafil in sildenafil non-responders: A multi-centre, double-blind, 12-233k, flexible-dose, placebo-controlled erectile dysfunction clinical trial. *BJU International* 2004; 94:1301–1309.

- Carson C, Rajfer J, Eardley I, et al. The efficacy and safety of tadalafil: an update. *BJU International* 2004; 93:1276–1281.

- Dasgupta R, Wiseman OJ, Kanabar G, Fowler CF, Mikol DD. Efficacy of sildenafil in the treatment of female sexual dysfunction due to multiple sclerosis. *J Urol* 2004; 171:1189–1193.

- Foley FW, LaRocca NG, Sanders AS, Zemon V. Rehabilitation of intimacy and sexual dysfunction in couples with multiple sclerosis. *Multiple Sclerosis* 2001; 7:417–421.

- Zorzon M, Zivadinov R, Bosco A, et al. Sexual dysfunction in multiple sclerosis: A case-control study. 1. Frequency and comparison of groups. *Multiple Sclerosis* 1999; 5:418–427.

Pain

- Archibald CJ, McGrath, PJ, Ritvo PG, et al. Pain prevalence, severity and impact in a clinic sample of multiple sclerosis patients. *Pain* 1994; 58:89–93.

- Berk C, Constantoyannis C, Honey CR. The treatment of trigeminal neuralgia in patients with multiple sclerosis using percutaneous radiofrequency rhizotomy. *Can J Neurol Sci* 2003; 30:320–323.

- Broggi G, Ferroli P, Franzini A, Servello D, Dones I. Microvascular decompression for trigeminal neuralgia: Comments on a series of 250 cases, including 10 patients with multiple sclerosis. *J Neurol Neurosurg Psychiatry* 2000; 68:59–64.

- DMKG Study group. Misoprostol In the treatment of trigeminal neuralgia associated with multiple sclerosis. *J Neurol* 2003; 250:542–545.

- Ehde DM, Gibbons LE, Chwastiak L, Bombardier CH, Sullivan MD, Kraft GH. Chronic pain in large community sample of persons with multiple sclerosis. *Multiple Sclerosis* 2003; 9:605–611.

- Eldridge PR, Sinha AK, Javadpour M, Littlechild P, Varma TR. Microvascular decompression for trigeminal neuralgia In patients with multiple sclerosis. *Stereotact Funct Neurosurg* 2003; 81:57–64.

- Khan OA. Gabapentin relieves trigeminal neuralgia in multiple sclerosis patients. *Neurology* 1998; 51:611–614.

- Svendsen KB, Jensen TS, Bach FW. Does the cannabinoid dronabinol reduce central pain in multiple sclerosis? Randomized double-blind placebo-controlled crossover trial. *Br Med J.* 2004; 329:253–256.

- Svendsen KB, Jensen TS, Overvad K, Hansen HJ, Koch-Henriksen N, Bach FW. Pain in patients with multiple sclerosis: A population-based study. *Arch Neurol* 2003; 60:1089–1094.

Cognitive Dysfunction

- Jonnsson A, Korfitzen EM, Heltberg A, Ravnborg MH, Byskov-Ottosen E. Effects of neuropsychological treatment in patients with multiple sclerosis. *Acta Neurol Scand* 1993; 88:394–400.

- Krupp LB, Christodoulou C, Melville P, Scherl WF, MacAllister WS, Elkins LE. Donepezil improved memory in multiple sclerosis in a randomized clinical trial. *Neurology* 2004; 63:1579–1585.

- Parry AM, Scott RB, Palace J, Smith S, Matthews PM. Potentially adaptive functional changes in cognitive processing for patients with multiple sclerosis and their acute modulation by rivistigmine. *Brain* 2003; 126:2750–1760.

- Plohmann AM, Kappos L, Ammann W, et al. Computer assisted retraining of attentional impairments in patients with multiple sclerosis. *J Neurol Neurosurg Psychiatry* 1998; 64:455–462.

- Solari A, Motta A, Mendozzi L, Pucci E, Forni M, Mancardi G, Pozzilli C. Computer-aided retraining of memory and attention in people with multiple sclerosis: A randomized double-blind controlled trial. *J Neurol Sci* 2004; 222:99–104.

Psychological and Psychiatric Dysfunction

- Feinstein A. The neuropsychiatry of multiple sclerosis. *Can J Psychiatry* 2004; 49:157–63.

- Feinstein A, Roy P, Lobaugh N, Feinstein K, O'Connor P, Black S. Structural brain abnormalities in multiple sclerosis patients with major depression. *Neurology* 2004; 62:586–90.

- Ron MA, Logsdail SJ. Psychiatric morbidity in multiple sclerosis: A clinical and MRI study. *Psychol Med* 1989; 19:887–895.

Other Symptoms

- Abraham S, Scheinberg LC, Smith CR, LaRocca NG. Neurologic impairment and disability status in outpatients with multiple sclerosis reporting dysphagia symptomatology. *J Neuro Rehab* 1997; 11(1):7–13.

- Howard RS, Wiles CM, Hirsch NP, et al. Respiratory involvement in multiple sclerosis. *Brain* 1992; 115: 479–494.

- Schwid SR, Petrie MD, Murray R et al. A randomized controlled study of the acute and chronic effects of cooling therapy for MS. *Neurology* 2003; 60:1955–1960.

- Starck M, Albrecht H, Pollmann W, Straube A, Dieterich M. Drug therapy for acquired pendular nystagmus in multiple sclerosis. *J Neurol* 1997; 244:9–16.

Neurorehabilitation

General Reviews

- European Multiple Sclerosis Platform. *Recommendations on Rehabilitation Services for Persons with Multiple Sclerosis in Europe.* Associazione Italiana Scelosi Multipla. Genoa Italy, October 2004.

- Freeman J, Ford H, Mattison P,Thompson AJ, Ridley J, Haffenden S. Developing MS Healthcare Standards: Evidence-Based Recommendations for Service Providers. MS Society of Great Britain and Northern Ireland, 2002.

- Thompson AJ. The effectiveness of neurological rehabilitation in multiple sclerosis. *J Rehabil Res Dev.* 2000; 37:455–461.

Outcome Measures

- Cella DF, Dineen K, Arnason B, et al. Validation of the functional assessment of multiple sclerosis quality of life instrument. *Neurology* 1996; 47(1):129–139.

- Fischer JS, LaRocca NG, Miller DM, et al. Recent developments in the assessment of quality of life in multiple sclerosis (MS). *Multiple Sclerosis* 1999; 5:251–260.

- Hobart JC, Lamping DL, Fitzpatrick R, Riazi A, Thompson AJ. The Multiple Sclerosis Impact Scale (MSIS-29): A new patient-based outcome measure. *Brain* 2001; 124:962–973.

- Hobart JC, Riazi A, Lamping DL, Fitzpatrick R, Thompson AJ. Measuring the impact of MS on walking ability: The 12-item MS Walking Scale (MSWS-12). *Neurology* 2003; 31–36.

- Jonsson A, Dock J, Ravnborg MH. Quality of life as a measure of rehabilitation outcome in patients with multiple sclerosis. *Acta Neurol Scand* 1996; 93:229–235.

- Rossiter DA, Edmondson A, Al-Shahi R, Thompson AJ. Integrated care pathways in multiple sclerosis: Completing the audit cycle. *Multiple Sclerosis* 1998; 4:85–89.

- Sharrack B, Hughes RAC, Soudain S, Dunn G. The psychometric properties of clinical rating scales used in multiple sclerosis. *Brain* 1999; 122:141–160.

- Thompson AJ, Hobart JC. Multiple sclerosis: Assessment of disability and disability scales. *J Neurol* 1998; 245(4):189–196.

- Vickrey BG, Hays RD, Harooni R, Myers LW, Ellison GW. A health-related quality of life measure for multiple sclerosis. *Qual Life Res* 1995; 4(3):187–206.

Diagnostic Phase

- McDonald WI, Compston A, Edan G, et al. Recommended diagnostic criteria for multiple sclerosis: Guidelines from the International Panel on the Diagnosis of Multiple Sclerosis. *Ann Neurol* 2001; 50:121–127.

- Porter B, Keenan E, Record E, Thompson AJ. Diagnosis of MS: A comparison of three different clinical settings. *Multiple Sclerosis* 2003; 9:431–439.

Minimal Disability

- Craig J, Young CA, Ennis M, Baker G, Boggild M. A randomized, controlled trial comparing rehabilitation against standard therapy in multiple sclerosis patients receiving intravenous steroid therapy treatment. *J Neurol, Neurosurg Psychiatry* 2003; 74:1225–1230.

- Liu C, Playford D, Thompson AJ. Does neurorehabilitation have a role in relapsing-remitting multiple sclerosis? *J Neurol* 2003; 250:1214–1218.

- Lublin FD, Baier M, Cutter G. Effect of relapses on the development of residual deficit in multiple sclerosis. *Neurology* 2003; 61:1528–1532.

- Mostert S, Kesselring J. Effects of short-term exercise training programme on aerobic fitness, fatigue, health perception and activity level of subjects with multiple sclerosis. *Multiple Sclerosis* 2002; 8:161–168.

- Petajan JH, Gappmaier E, White AT, et al. Impact of aerobic training on fitness and quality of life in multiple sclerosis. *Ann Neurol* 1996; 39(4):432–441.

- Romberg A, Virtanen A, Aunola S, Karppi S. Exercise capacity, disability and leisure physical activity of subjects with multiple sclerosis. *Multiple Sclerosis* 2004; 10:212–218.

- Wiles CM, Newcombe RG, Fuller KJ, et al. A controlled, randomized, crossover trial of the effects of physiotherapy on mobility on chronic multiple sclerosis. *J Neurol Neurosurg Psychiatry* 2001; 70:174–179.

Moderate Disability

- Aisen ML, Sevilla D, Fox N. Inpatient rehabilitation for multiple sclerosis. *J Neuro Rehab* 1996; 10:43–46.

- Di Fabio RP, Soderberg J, Choi T, Hansen CR, Schapiro RT. Extended outpatient rehabilitation: Its influence on symptom frequency, fatigue and functional status for persons with progressive multiple sclerosis. *Arch Phys Med Rehabil* 1998; 79(2):141–146.

- Freeman JA, Langdon DW, Hobart JC, Thompson AJ. Inpatient rehabilitation in multiple sclerosis: Do the benefits carry over into the community? *Neurology* 1999; 52:50–56.

- Freeman JA, Langdon DW, Hobart JC, Thompson AJ. The impact of inpatient rehabilitation on progressive multiple sclerosis. *Ann Neurol* 1997; 42(2):236–244.

- Grasso MG, Troisi E, Rizzi F, Morelli D, Paolucci S. Prognostic factors in multidisciplinary rehabilitation in multiple sclerosis: An outcome study. *Multiple Sclerosis*, 2005; 11:719–724.

- Jonsson A, Ravnborg MH. Rehabilitation in multiple sclerosis. *Phys Rehab Med* 1998; 10(1):75–100.

- Langdon DW, Thompson AJ. Multiple sclerosis: A preliminary study of selected variables affecting rehabilitation outcome. *Multiple Sclerosis* 1999; 5:94–100.

- Patti F, Ciancio MR, Cacopardo M, Reggio E, Fiorilla T, Palermo F, Reggio A, Thompson AJ. Effects of a short outpatient rehabilitation treatment on disability of multiple sclerosis patients. A randomized controlled trial. *J Neurol* 2003; 250:861–866.

- Romberg A, Virtanens A, Ruutiainen J et al. Effects of a six-month exercise programme on patients with multiple sclerosis. *Neurol* 2004; 63:2034–2038.

- Solari A, Filippini G, Gasco P, et al. Physical rehabilitation has a positive effect on disability in multiple sclerosis patients. *Neurology* 1999; 52(1):57–62.

- Storr L, Sorenson PS, Ravnborg M. The efficacy of multidisciplinary rehabilitation in stable multiple sclerosis patients *Multiple Sclerosis* (in press).

Severe Disability

- Gruenewald DA, Higginson IJ, Vivat B, Edmonds P, Burman RE. Quality of life measures for the palliative care of people severely affected by multiple sclerosis: A systematic review. *Multiple Sclerosis* 2004; 10:690–704.

Models of Care

- Carton H, Loos R, Pacolet J, Versieck K, Vlietink R. Utilisation and cost of professional care and assistance according to disability of patients with multiple sclerosis in Flanders (Belgium). *J Neurol Neurosurg, Psychiatry* 1998; 64:444–450.

- Freeman JA, Thompson AJ. Community services in multiple sclerosis: Still a matter of chance. *J Neurol, Neurosurg, Psychiatry* 2000; 69:728–732.

- Pozzilli C, Brunetti M, Amicosante AMV et al. Home based management in multiple sclerosis: Results of a randomized controlled trial. *J Neurol, Neurosurg and Psychiatry* 2002; 73:250–255.

Chapter 5

Unconventional Therapies and MS

The previous chapters of this book primarily review conventional medical therapies for MS. In this chapter, unconventional medical therapies are considered. These unconventional therapies are important to review because many people with MS and other chronic diseases are interested in and use these therapies. Among unconventional therapies, there is much variability in the quality of the available information and also in the effectiveness, safety, and cost of the therapies. Consequently, it is especially important to be knowledgeable and cautious in this area. This chapter provides background information about unconventional medicine, strategies for evaluating unconventional therapies, and MS-specific information about unconventional therapies that are popular or are particularly relevant to MS.

DEFINITION OF UNCONVENTIONAL MEDICINE

Unconventional medicine is a term that is surprisingly difficult to define. Part of the difficulty is that many different terms are used in this area. In addition to *unconventional medicine,* other frequently used terms include *alternative medicine, complementary medicine,* and *integrative medicine.*

117

One of the more commonly used terms is *unconventional medicine*. This is sometimes defined as therapies that are not typically taught in medical schools or generally available in hospitals. However, this definition is awkward because it states what unconventional medicine *is not* as opposed to what it *is*. Also, this definition is a "moving target" because it depends on the medical traditions of the country in which it is used, and in some countries, including the United States, many medical schools now offer courses in unconventional medicine.

There are many other definitions of unconventional medicine. One definition that is more precise, but also more complex, is provided by the National Institutes of Health (NIH). In this definition, unconventional medicine is subdivided into categories. These categories, with representative examples, include:

- Biologically based therapies: dietary supplements, diets, bee venom therapy

- Mind–body therapies: guided imagery, hypnosis, meditation

- Alternative medical systems: traditional Chinese medicine, Ayurveda, homeopathy

- Manipulative and body-based therapies: chiropractic, reflexology, massage

- Energy therapies: therapeutic touch, magnets

Other terms that are used refer to the way in which the therapies are used. Unconventional therapies that are used instead of conventional medicine are known as *alternative medicine*, while unconventional therapies that are used in conjunction with conventional medicine are called *complementary medicine*. A broader term is *complementary and alternative medicine*, which is often shortened to the acronym *CAM*. An even broader term, *integrative medicine,* refers to the combined use of conventional and unconventional medicine.

POPULARITY OF UNCONVENTIONAL MEDICINE

There have been many studies of the use of CAM in the general population. One well-known study identified the popularity of CAM and stimulated interest in the subject. This United States study, reported by Dr. David Eisenberg and others in 1997, found that about 40 percent of people used some form of CAM and that people visited unconventional medical practitioners more frequently than primary care physicians. Almost 20 percent of people were taking prescription medication along with some type of herb, vitamin, or other dietary supplement. Nearly one-half used CAM without the advice of a CAM practitioner or physician, and more than one-half (60 percent) did not discuss their use of unconventional medicine with their physician.

CAM use in people with MS appears to be greater than that in the general population. In studies in several countries, including the United States, Canada, the Netherlands, Germany, and Australia, it has been found that about one-half to three-fourths of people with MS use some form of unconventional medicine. In these studies, nearly all people with MS use unconventional medicine in conjunction with conventional medicine. In other words, the unconventional medicine is used as *complementary medicine.* Some of the CAM therapies that are more commonly used by people with MS include special diets, dietary supplements, prayer and spirituality, chiropractic medicine, and massage.

EVIDENCE FOR THE SAFETY AND EFFECTIVENESS OF THERAPIES

Different types of evidence may be available to determine the safety and effectiveness of unconventional as well as conventional therapies. When considering a therapy, it is extremely important to understand these different levels of evidence and how they apply specifically to MS. Information about a therapy may be based on theoretical arguments, experimental studies, or clinical trials of people with MS. (Chapter 1 includes a detailed review of the different types of evidence that may be available for a particular therapy.)

When reviewing information about a therapy, it is important to determine the strength of the evidence that is available. Some CAM literature does not distinguish between the various levels of evidence or makes very strong recommendations on the basis of weak evidence. For example, a CAM therapy such as a dietary supplement might be highly recommended for MS because it suppresses the immune system, produces therapeutic effects in the animal model of MS, and has minimal side effects. Although this sounds promising, there is no clinical trial evidence. As a result, it is quite likely that this therapy would not be an effective treatment for MS.

It is important to recognize that among all of the conventional and unconventional therapies that are claimed to alter the disease course in MS the best evidence that is currently available is that which has been obtained for the conventional medications that are in widespread use, including interferon beta-1a (Avonex®, Rebif®), interferon beta-1b (Betaseron®, Betaferon®), glatiramer acetate (Copaxone®), and mitoxantrone (Novantrone®). There are no CAM therapies that have a similar level of evidence to support their use as these disease-modifying medications.

Ideally, there should be high quality clinical evidence for well-tolerated therapies that could cure MS and completely eliminate all MS symptoms. Unfortunately this is not the case. As has been described in other chapters of this book, there have been remarkable advances recently in conventional medicine in treating MS. However, there is no cure for the disease, and the disease-modifying and symptomatic conventional therapies that are available are often only partially effective or may produce side effects. Due to this situation and in an effort "to do the best we can," there are circumstances in which conventional medicine uses approaches that are not entirely proven. These approaches must be used thoughtfully and with recognition of the limited evidence. There must be careful weighing of possible risks and benefits. Examples of these unconventional approaches include assessing the effectiveness of disease-modifying therapies by subjective clinical and MRI criteria, using unproven "combination therapies" to try to modify disease course, and using symptomatic therapies for which there is limited clinical evidence ("off-label" use).

These limitations of conventional medicine are part of the reason that some people with MS are interested in CAM. For people with MS who are interested in CAM, there should be a careful and thoughtful approach that is similar to that used for conventional therapies for which the information is limited. It is important to obtain unbiased MS-relevant information, determine the safety and effectiveness of the therapy, and discuss the therapy with a physician or other conventional health care provider. If the therapy is pursued, there should be a plan for monitoring for a response. If that response does not occur, then the therapy should be discontinued and other approaches should be considered. It is important to use caution, realize that the safety and effectiveness information about most CAM therapies is limited, and recognize that there is a certain degree of risk that an individual takes in pursuing CAM.

USING UNCONVENTIONAL MEDICINE

If a decision is made to consider unconventional therapies, there are some guidelines that may be especially helpful. These guidelines have broad applications to a variety of unconventional therapies.

First, it is important to know when it may be reasonable to use CAM. For example, it might be reasonable to consider CAM for symptoms such as mild fatigue or mild muscle stiffness. Also, it may be reasonable to use CAM for conditions for which conventional medicine has no effective therapies or only partially effective therapies. On the other hand, there are situations in which CAM is inappropriate. Severe conditions, such as disabling muscle stiffness or severe pain, or a serious disease, such as MS, should not be treated initially or exclusively with CAM therapies. In some of these situations, it may be reasonable for people who are interested in CAM to use CAM along with conventional medicine.

Some CAM books make erroneous claims about MS, some of which are potentially dangerous. One relatively frequent misunderstanding is that MS is an immune disease and that, consequently, it should be treated by stimulating the immune system with dietary supplements. *This is incorrect.* MS is an immune disease, but it is generally characterized by excessive immune system activity. As a result, effective MS therapies generally *decrease* immune system activity.

There are features of some CAM therapies that should raise concerns, including:

- "Secret ingredients" or little objective information about safety or effectiveness

- Extremely strong claims about effectiveness, such as claims that a single therapy is effective for many different conditions

- Use of "testimonials" in which individuals make very strong claims about effectiveness

- Much cost or effort is involved, such as inpatient therapy or intravenous treatment

There are common misconceptions about dietary supplements, which includes vitamins, minerals, and herbs. Some supplements are claimed to have therapeutic effects and no side effects. This is not true. Supplements, especially herbs, are similar to medications and contain chemicals that may produce beneficial effects but may also cause side effects. Also, it is sometimes claimed that "more is better," especially with vitamins and minerals. This is not correct and may actually be dangerous. High doses of many supplements may produce side effects. Finally, it is sometimes stated that natural compounds are safe and beneficial. In fact, there are many products that are natural but are also very toxic. Examples include mercury, arsenic, animal venoms, and poisonous mushrooms.

UNCONVENTIONAL THERAPIES RELEVANT TO MS

There are limitations with information about CAM therapies, and caution should be used in considering these therapies. At the same time, for some individuals the thoughtful use of CAM therapies, especially in combination with conventional medicine, may allow for an individualized treatment plan and provide hope, control, and a sense of empowerment. The remainder of this chapter will provide MS-relevant information about CAM therapies that have been specifically studied in MS, that are used commonly in the general population or by people with MS, or that raise specific safety concerns (Table 5-1). Some of the unconventional therapies used by people with MS include:

Acupuncture and Traditional Chinese Medicine

Description: Acupuncture is one component of traditional Chinese medicine (TCM). Other components include traditional Chinese herbs, nutrition, exercise, stress reduction, and massage. TCM is based on a theory of body function that is very different from that of Western medicine. Specifically, it is believed that energy, or *qi*, flows through 14 major pathways, or *meridians*, on the body. There is also a balance of opposites, which are known as *yin* and *yang*. According to TCM, disease occurs when there is disturbance or disharmony of energy. With acupuncture, thin, metallic needles are inserted in specific points on the meridians.

Rationale: From the perspective of TCM, it is believed that the insertion of acupuncture needles alters the flow of energy in

Table 5-1. Unconventional Therapies

Acupuncture and traditional Chinese medicine
Bee venom therapy
Cannabis (marijuana)
Chiropractic medicine
Cooling therapy
Dental amalgam removal
Dietary supplements
    −antioxidants
    −cranberry and other supplements used for urinary tract infections
    −echinacea and other "immune-stimulating" supplements
    −ginkgo biloba
    −kava kava
    −Padma 28
    −psyllium
    −St. John's wort
    −valerian
    −vitamin B_{12}
    −vitamin D and calcium
    −zinc
Diets
    −Swank diet
    −supplementation with omega-6 fatty acids
    −supplementation with omega-3 fatty acids
Feldenkrais
Guided imagery and relaxation
Hyperbaric oxygen
Magnetic field therapy (electromagnetic therapy)
Massage
Neural therapy
Reflexology
Tai chi
Yoga

---

such a way that it produces therapeutic effects. From a Western scientific perspective, the mechanism by which acupuncture might produce its effects is not clear. Acupuncture may alter activity in specific brain regions or lead to the release of specific chemicals, such as serotonin or pain-relieving *opioids.*

Evaluation: There is limited information about acupuncture in people with MS. Two recent preliminary studies indicate that 20–25 percent of people with MS have tried acupuncture. Two older studies reported beneficial effects of acupuncture in people with MS, but these findings are not definitive because the studies were small and not rigorously designed. A more recent preliminary study suggests that acupuncture may improve the symptoms of MS-related bladder dysfunction. In people who do not have MS, several studies indicate that acupuncture improves pain, nausea, and vomiting. Studies of Chinese herbal medicine in MS are also limited. Some studies, published in Chinese, report that Chinese herbal therapy decreases the attack rate and slows the progression of the disease. These studies are difficult to evaluate because they are not available in English.

Risks/costs: Acupuncture is usually well tolerated, especially when it is done by a well-trained acupuncturist. Sterile needles should be used to avoid infections, including hepatitis and AIDS. Acupuncture is moderately expensive. The safety of Chinese herbal medicine has not been well characterized, especially in people with MS. There is a theoretical risk of worsening MS with immune-stimulating herbs, which include Asian ginseng, astragalus, and maitake and reishi mushrooms. In addition, one herb that mildly suppresses the immune system, Thunder God Vine, or *Tripterygium wilfordii*, may produce serious side effects, including death. Chinese herbal medicine is a low cost therapy.

In the opinion of the Committee, there is no definitive evidence to support the use of acupuncture in MS. There are studies suggesting that it may be alleviate some

MS-related symptoms, especially pain. Further study is needed to determine if acupuncture has any definitive therapeutic effects in MS. Acupuncture is a low risk, moderately expensive therapy. Chinese herbal medicine is a low cost therapy that is of unknown effectiveness in MS. There are risks associated with the use of some Chinese herbal therapies.

Bee Venom Therapy

Description: Bee venom therapy (BVT) is one form of apitherapy, a term used to describe the use of bees or bee products to treat medical conditions. Apitherapy was used in ancient Egypt and ancient Greece. Areas of recent interest in BVT include MS and arthritis. In BVT, tweezers are used to place bees on particular body parts. Typically, there are three treatment sessions each week, and each session involves 20–40 stings.

Rationale: There are several theoretical explanations for a beneficial effect of BVT in MS. One explanation is that the inflammation of the bee sting causes the body to produce an anti-inflammatory response. This response is then thought to act towards the sting but also towards other inflammatory conditions, which could include MS or arthritis. Recent studies suggest that the chemical components of bee venom inhibit an enzyme (cyclo-oxygenase 2) and the production of proteins (tumor necrosis factor-alpha, interleukin-1beta) involved in inflammation. Finally, apamin, a bee venom constituent, inhibits the actions of proteins on cells known as *potassium channels*. This is similar to the effects of 4-aminopyridine (4AP), a conventional medication that may decrease MS-related fatigue. It is not known whether blood or nervous system levels of the venom are high enough after a sting to produce any of these biochemical effects.

Evaluation: Clinical studies of BVT are limited. The preliminary report of a study in the animal model of MS found that BVT was ineffective or may actually have produced worsening relative to placebo-treated animals. A safety study of BVT in humans was conducted at Georgetown University in the United States. The results of this study have not been published.

Risks/costs: BVT is usually well tolerated. Very rarely, bee stings may cause anaphylaxis, a severe and potentially fatal allergic reaction. It is sometimes recommended that bee stings be given around the eye for people with MS-related visual problems. This practice should be avoided because bee stings in this area may actually cause optic neuritis, an inflammation of the optic nerve that is associated with MS. BVT is a low-moderate cost therapy.

In the opinion of the Committee, bee venom therapy has not been adequately studied in MS. There is no evidence that it produces therapeutic effects. It is of low-moderate cost and may rarely produce severe side effects.

Cannabis (Marijuana)

Description: For years, it has been claimed that cannabis, also known as *marijuana*, is an effective treatment for MS (see also "Spasticity" section of Chapter 4). Cannabis, which is illegal in many countries, contains compounds known as cannabinoids. These compounds, which include tetrahydrocannabinol (THC), produce specific biochemical effects in the body. Cannabis may be smoked or ingested. There are prescription medications that contain cannabinoids. In the United States, THC is available as dronabinol (Marinol®). In Europe, Canada, and Australia, a synthetic form of THC is available as nabilone (Cesamet®).

Rationale: Cannabinoids exert several biological effects that, on a theoretical basis, could be therapeutic for MS. First, they bind to proteins in the central nervous system (CB1 receptors) that suppress excessive nerve cell activity. This could, on a theoretical basis, decrease some MS symptoms such as pain and muscle stiffness (spasticity). Also, cannabinoids bind to another type of protein on immune cells (CB2 receptors) and mildly suppress the immune system. It is possible that cannabinoids are able to slow down the disease process in MS through this mechanism. Finally, cannabinoids may protect against nerve cell injury by decreasing the damage caused by free radicals and "excitotoxicity," an injurious form of excitatory nerve cell activity.

Evaluation: Studies of the effects of cannabis on MS and experimental allergic encephalomyelitis (EAE), the animal model of MS, are limited and inconclusive. In EAE, some symptoms, including spasticity and tremor, are improved with cannabinoid treatment. In addition, high doses of cannabinoids decrease the overall severity of EAE. There are mixed results in studies of the actual disease in humans. In several surveys of people with MS who have smoked cannabis, symptoms commonly reported to be improved include pain, spasticity, depression, and anxiety. Importantly, surveys such as this are not rigorous enough to provide definitive evidence for effectiveness. Actual clinical studies of the effects of smoked or oral cannabis on MS symptoms are of variable quality. Some, but not all, of these studies have found improvement in spasticity. A 1999 review by the National Academy of Sciences/Institute of Medicine (NAS/IOM) stated that there was suggestive evidence that smoked and oral cannabis may alleviate MS-related spasticity. In 2003, the results of the first large formal clinical trial of an extract of cannabis and oral THC on MS symptoms were reported. For a variety of MS symptoms, there was no therapeutic effect as determined by objective tests based on clinical exams. However, subjective benefits, as reported by people in the study, were found for spasticity, pain, and sleep quality. In a 12-month follow-up to this study, THC showed a small treatment effect on muscle spasticity, and there was a suggestion of a therapeutic effect on disability, especially in the THC-treated group. In the United Kingdom, there are plans to conduct a long-term clinical trial of cannabinoid use in progressive MS. The effects of cannabis on the immune system and on disease activity in MS are not clear. Contrary to what one might expect, one study found that cannabinoids actually produced immune-stimulating effects.

Risks/costs: There are significant risks associated with smoking cannabis, including nausea, vomiting, sedation, increased risk of seizures, and poor pregnancy outcomes. Driving may be impaired for up to 8 hours after smoking cannabis. High doses of cannabis may impair heart function, decrease reaction time, and produce coordination and visual difficulties. Chronic cannabis use may cause heart attacks, impair lung function, cause dependence and apathy, and increase the risk of cancer of the lung, head, and neck. Smoked cannabis and prescription medications containing cannabinoids are of low-moderate cost.

In the opinion of the Committee, additional research is needed to determine if cannabis is safe or effective in MS. Some experimental and clinical studies suggest that cannabis may alleviate some MS symptoms and may decrease the severity of the disease. However, there is no definitive evidence for a therapeutic effect, there are significant risks associated with cannabis, and cannabis is illegal in many countries.

Chiropractic Medicine

Description: Chiropractic medicine is one of the most popular forms of CAM in the United States, which may relate to the fact that this therapy was founded in the United States. Chiropractic medicine is based on the concept that the nervous system plays a critical role in health and that many diseases are caused by abnormal pressure of bones on the nerves in the spine. Manipulation of the spine is an important component of chiropractic care. There are two groups of chiropractors. "Straights" only use spinal manipulation, while "mixers" use manipulation along with other therapies, including dietary recommendations, herb and vitamin supplements, ultrasound, and massage.

Rationale: Chiropractors believe that subluxations, misalignments of the bones of the spine, cause abnormal pressure on the nerves that travel from the spinal cord to the muscles and organs of the body. It is claimed that this abnormal pressure results in impaired muscle and organ function. Treatment involves spinal manipulation techniques, known as "adjustments," which are thought to normalize bone positions and restore normal function.

Evaluation: There are no well-designed studies that document that spinal manipulation or other chiropractic methods can alter the disease course in MS. Isolated clinical reports have described improvement in some MS symptoms with chiropractic treatment, but there are no systematic clinical studies of chiropractic treatment for MS symptoms. In studies of other conditions, it has been found that spinal manipulation may decrease low back pain. However, these studies are of variable quality. The effectiveness of chiropractic treatment for chronic neck pain and headache is not clear.

Risks/costs: Chiropractic treatment is generally well tolerated. Between 1900 and 1980, 135 complications were reported in the medical literature. One of the more common adverse effects is achy muscles, which may be present for 1 to 2 days after manipulation. A rare but serious complication associated with neck manipulation is stroke. Very rarely, low back manipulation may cause compression of the nerves of the lower spine ("cauda equine syndrome"). Bone and disc injuries of the spine are uncommon with spine manipulation. Pregnant women, people taking anticoagulant medications, and people with spinal bone fractures, spine trauma, significant disc herniations, bone cancer or infection, severe osteoporosis, and severe arthritis should avoid chiropractic therapy. Importantly, since chiropractors are not as well trained in diagnosis as physicians, people with serious diseases or conditions should be evaluated and treated by a physician and should not substitute chiropractic medicine for conventional medicine. Chiropractic therapy is of low-moderate cost.

*In the opinion of the Committee there are no well-de-
signed studies that demonstrate that chiropractic spinal
manipulation or other forms of chiropractic therapy alter the course of MS or are beneficial for MS-specific
symptoms. Spinal manipulation may be effective for low
back pain. Chiropractic therapy is of low-moderate cost
and, although associated with very rare but serious side
effects, it is usually well tolerated.*

Cooling Therapy

Description: Cooling therapy is a form of CAM that is unique
to MS (see also Chapter 4). It has been known for years that
changes in body temperature may significantly affect MS symptoms. Specifically, small increases in body temperature (0.5°
C) may worsen symptoms, while small decreases may improve
symptoms. Consequently, various cooling methods have been
developed. These methods range from simple techniques, such
as drinking cold liquids and staying in air-conditioned areas, to
complex methods, such as using specially designed cooling suits.
Cooling suits may be *passive* or *active*. Passive garments use
evaporation or ice packs for cooling; active garments use circu-
lating coolants.

Rationale: In MS, there is damage to myelin, the insulating
layer of the nerve fiber that facilitates the conduction of nerve
impulses. In these injured nerves, conduction of signals is
blocked with small increases in temperature. Conversely, small
decreases in temperature may facilitate transmission of signals.

Evaluation: Beneficial effects of cooling garments have been
noted in several clinical studies. Unfortunately, some of these
reports are preliminary and most of the studies have been small
and not rigorously conducted. Among these studies, improvement in fatigue is frequently seen. Other symptoms showing
improvement include leg strength, spasticity, walking, bladder
dysfunction, sexual difficulties, visual changes, speech difficult-

ies, cognitive difficulties, and incoordination. The results of the most rigorous cooling study in MS (randomized, controlled, blinded) have been published recently. In this study, it was found that, on the basis of objective measures, cooling was associated with mildly improved walking and visual function. By subjective measures, cooling improved fatigue, strength, and cognition. Cooling garments may be especially well suited for those who are known to be heat-sensitive.

Risks/costs: The use of cooling garments is usually well tolerated. Some people feel uncomfortable when cooling begins, and handling of the garments may be cumbersome. Some people with MS have a paradoxical sensitivity to cold, in which case cooling may actually *worsen* symptoms. Costs of cooling are dependent on the method used. Simple techniques are of low cost. Cooling garments are of moderate cost. Passive garments are generally less expensive than active garments.

In the opinion of the Committee, cooling is a low risk and relatively inexpensive therapy that has a clear scientific rationale. It is possibly effective for treating some MS symptoms, especially fatigue. Further studies are needed to determine whether it is definitely effective.

Dental Amalgam Removal

Description: Removal of dental amalgam has been proposed as a treatment method for MS. For more than 150 years, cavities have been filled with dental amalgam, which is composed of mercury as well as silver, copper, tin, and zinc. Amalgam is currently used in about 80–90 percent of tooth restorations.

Rationale: Through various mechanisms, it is claimed that amalgam causes or worsens MS and many other diseases. The small levels of solid mercury and mercury vapor that are released from amalgam are believed to damage the immune system and nervous system. Also, it is claimed that MS is caused by electrical currents that are generated by mercury or by allergic reactions to mercury. Treatment involves removal of the amalgam and replacement with gold or plastic fillings.

Evaluation: There are anecdotal reports of people with MS experiencing beneficial effects with amalgam removal. However, there is no evidence that mercury causes MS or that removal of dental amalgam improves the course of MS. Brain mercury levels are not higher in people with MS than in the general population. MS occurred as a disease prior to the routine use of amalgam in dental practice, and there are people with MS who have no dental amalgam. In some epidemiological studies, there has been a trend toward people with MS having more dental amalgam exposure. However, these findings have not been statistically significant. An important observation with regard to amalgam removal is that mercury intake from amalgam represents only 10 percent or less of the total mercury consumed by a person. Other major sources of mercury are food (especially fish), pollution, paints, disinfectants, and medications. Dental amalgam removal as a treatment for MS is not supported by multiple professional organizations, including the National MS Society of the United States.

Risks/costs: Dental amalgam removal is generally well tolerated. Rarely, it may damage tooth structure or nerves. For a short time after amalgam removal, there may be an *increase* in blood mercury levels. Amalgam removal is moderately expensive.

In the opinion of the Committee, dental amalgam removal is a moderately expensive, generally well-tolerated procedure. However, there is no evidence that mercury from amalgam causes MS or that removal of amalgam has a beneficial effect on MS symptoms or on the course of MS.

Dietary Supplements

A wide range of compounds is included in the category of dietary supplements. Vitamins and minerals are commonly used supplements. Herbs are also widely used in some countries. Other diverse compounds, including amino acids, hormones, and enzymes, are also classified as dietary supplements. In this section, dietary supplements will be considered that are popular or are relevant to MS.

Antioxidants

Description: Free radicals are chemicals that may injure cells in the body through a process known as *oxidative damage.* Antioxidants are compounds that can decrease oxidative damage. Commonly used antioxidants include selenium and vitamins A, C, and E. Other compounds in the antioxidant category include alpha-lipoic acid, inosine, uric acid, coenzyme Q10 (CoQ10), grape seed extract, pycnogenol, and oligomeric proanthocyanidins ("OPCs"). Antioxidants are sometimes specifically marketed as a treatment for MS.

Rationale: There are two major reasons that antioxidants are relevant to MS. First, free radicals may be involved in the pathology of MS. Myelin, the *insulation* of nerve fibers, may be injured in MS by the release of free radicals by immune cells. Also, the nerve fibers themselves, the axons, are damaged in MS through a degenerative process that may involve free radicals. Indeed, some studies indicate that oxidative damage is increased in EAE, the animal model of MS, and in tissue from people with MS. The other MS-relevant aspect of antioxidants is that diets that are enriched in polyunsaturated fatty acids, which are sometimes recommended for MS (see "Diets"), may cause vitamin E deficiency and supplementation with vitamin E may be needed.

Evaluation: Specific studies of antioxidants in MS are very limited. Studies in EAE, the animal model of MS, indicate that antioxidants may decrease disease severity. Recent studies have shown that alpha-lipoic acid and uric acid are effective therapies for EAE. In a human study, it was found that 18 people with MS who were treated for 5 weeks with vitamin C, vitamin E, and selenium did not experience any adverse effects. This study was too small and too short to provide any definitive results about the safety and effectiveness of antioxidants in MS. Clinical studies in people with MS are currently being conducted with alpha-lipoic acid and inosine, a compound that is converted to uric acid.

Risks/costs: Many antioxidant compounds activate immune cells known as *T cells* and macrophages. Since these cells are already excessively active in MS, further stimulation by antioxidants could potentially worsen the disease. Whether this occurs and is clinically important in MS has not been investigated. Thus, it represents a *theoretical risk.* The safety of many dietary supplements, including antioxidants, has not been determined in women who are pregnant or breastfeeding. Supplementation with antioxidants is a low-cost therapy.

In the opinion of the Committee, there is theoretical and experimental evidence that antioxidants could be of therapeutic value in MS. However, there are no well-designed clinical studies that have addressed whether antioxidants are indeed effective or safe in MS. Further clinical studies of antioxidants in people with MS are needed and are currently underway. Antioxidants are inexpensive and are associated with theoretical risks in MS.

Cranberry and Other Supplements Used for Urinary Tract Infections

Description: People with MS are prone to bladder difficulties, including urinary tract infections (UTIs). Cranberry, derived from the fruit of the cranberry plant, may prevent urinary tract infections.

Rationale: In the past, it was thought that cranberry might prevent UTIs by making the urine acidic. This does not appear to be the case. Instead, two chemical constituents of cranberry, a type of sugar known as *fructose* and another compound known as *proanthocyanidin*, appear to keep bacteria from adhering to the wall of the urinary tract. Like antibiotic medications, cranberry may also kill some bacteria.

Evaluation: Limited clinical studies with cranberry indicate that it may prevent UTIs in some people. Specifically, beneficial effects have been found in studies of UTI prevention in women with normal bladder function. However, in limited studies of people with abnormal bladder function, which may occur in MS, cranberry was actually found to be ineffective for preventing UTIs. The ideal clinical trial with cranberry has not been done in any group of people. Due to the availability of antibiotic medications and the complications that may occur with UTIs in people with MS, known infections should be treated with antibiotics and not cranberry. The evidence for two other UTI-related dietary supplements, vitamin C and bearberry (uva-ursi), is less clear than that for cranberry. Clinical studies do not provide strong support for either of these in the prevention of UTIs. In addition, there is concern about bearberry because it contains hydroquinones, which are chemicals that may have cancer-causing properties.

Risks/costs: Cranberry is inexpensive and generally well tolerated. Cranberry tablets are less expensive than juice. Cranberry may interfere with blood-thinning medications, which include warfarin (Coumadin®). Long-term use of high doses may increase the risk of kidney stones and may cause gastrointestinal discomfort, loose stools, and nausea. There is insufficient information about the safety of cranberry in women who are pregnant or breastfeeding.

In the opinion of the Committee, cranberry is possibly effective for preventing UTIs in women with normal bladder function. In people with abnormal bladder function, cranberry does not appear to be effective for UTI prevention. Further clinical studies are needed to determine if

*it is definitely effective for UTI prevention in any group
of people. Cranberry should not be used to treat known
UTIs, especially in people with MS. It is usually well
tolerated and is inexpensive.*

Echinacea and Other "Immune-Stimulating" Supplements

Description: Echinacea and several other dietary supplements
are known to activate the immune system.

Rationale: In some alternative medicine books, it is erroneously
stated that MS is an immune disease and that, consequently,
people with MS should take echinacea and other dietary supplements that stimulate the immune system. This is incorrect and
potentially dangerous information. MS is an immune disease,
but it is generally characterized by excess immune system activity. Thus, most effective MS therapies decrease immune system
activity. Compounds that stimulate the immune system, such as
echinacea, could actually *worsen* the disease.

Evaluation: The immune system effects of some dietary supplements have undergone limited investigation. Generally, these
studies have focused on *test-tube* or animal model experiments.
These studies have investigated macrophages and T cells, components of the immune system that are excessively active in MS.
Activation of these cells has been produced by echinacea and
several other dietary supplements, including:

- Herbs: alfalfa, Asian ginseng, astragalus, cat's claw, gar-
  lic, maitake mushroom, mistletoe, shiitake mushroom,
  Siberian ginseng, stinging nettle

- Vitamins and minerals: antioxidant vitamins and minerals
  (see "Dietary Supplements: Antioxidants"), zinc

- Others: melatonin

Based on scientific evidence, these compounds pose theoretical risks to people with MS. Clinical studies of the effects of
these compounds on people with MS are not currently available,

and probably never will be. There is one report of a person who developed an MS-like disease (acute disseminated encephalomyelitis) after the injection of an herbal mixture that included echinacea.

Risks/costs: As noted, immune-stimulating compounds pose theoretical risks to people with MS. For echinacea specifically, it may accentuate the liver toxicity of some medications, which include some MS medications such as interferons and methotrexate. Immune-stimulating dietary supplements are of low-moderate cost.

In the opinion of the Committee, there is no documented benefit for echinacea and other immune-stimulating dietary supplements in MS. These compounds, which are of low-moderate cost, actually pose theoretical risks to people with MS.

Ginkgo Biloba

Description: Ginkgo biloba usually refers to the extract that is derived from the leaf of the ginkgo biloba tree. Among herbs, ginkgo is one of the most extensively studied and one of the most popular.

Rationale: There are several effects of ginkgo that are relevant to MS. First, it is possible that it could treat the disease itself. Ginkgo has antiinflammatory and anti-oxidant effects, both of which could be therapeutic for MS. In addition, since ginkgo may improve cognitive function in people with Alzheimer's disease, it has been proposed that it may have similar effects on MS-related cognitive dysfunction.

Evaluation: Ginkgo has undergone limited investigation in MS. Ginkgo and related compounds decreased disease severity in some but not all studies in the animal model of MS. One small study of people with MS found that it may be helpful for MS attacks, however this was *not* supported by a subsequent study that was larger and was more rigorously conducted. Thus, it does not appear to be effective for MS attacks. Whether ginkgo prevents attacks—in a way similar to interferons, glatiramer acetate, mitoxantrone, and natalizumab—has never been investigated. One preliminary study found that ginkgo may improve MS-related cognitive difficulties. Further studies are needed to determine if ginkgo has the effect of slowing the course of MS or improving MS cognitive difficulties. Studies are currently underway to evaluate the effects of ginkgo on cognitive function in MS.

Risks/costs: Ginkgo is usually well tolerated. It may have a blood-thinning effect and thus should be avoided in people who have bleeding disorders, take antiplatelet or anticoagulant medication, or are undergoing surgery. In addition, ginkgo may provoke seizures and should be used with caution by those with seizure disorders. It may also cause dizziness, rashes, headache, and gastrointestinal complaints, including nausea, vomiting, diarrhea, and flatulence. The safety of ginkgo in women who are pregnant or breastfeeding is not known. Ginkgo is inexpensive.

Ginkgo is a low-cost therapy that is usually well tolerated. Rarely, it may cause bleeding and provoke seizures. There is a rationale for its use as a disease-modifying therapy in MS and for MS-related cognitive dysfunction. However, there is very limited clinical evidence. It does not appear to be effective for treating MS attacks. One preliminary study found that it may be helpful for MS-associated cognitive difficulties; further studies in this area are needed.

Kava Kava

Description: Kava kava is derived from the root of the kava plant. For hundreds of years, it has been used medicinally and recreationally in the islands of the South Pacific. It was first used in Europe in the early 19th century, primarily for treating venereal diseases. Its primary use now is for anxiety, which may occur in people with MS.

Rationale: Kava kava contains compounds known as *kavapyrones* or *kavalactones*. These compounds interact with specific proteins in the brain known as *GABA-A receptors*. These are the same proteins that mediate the actions of some anti-anxiety drugs, which including diazepam (Valium®) and clonazepam (Klonopin®).

Evaluation: On the basis of several clinical trials of kava kava, this herb may be an effective therapy for mild anxiety. It is probably *not* effective for more severe forms of anxiety. It is sometimes claimed to be an effective treatment for insomnia, but it has only undergone limited study for this condition.

Risks/costs: In the past, kava kava was considered a generally safe herb. However, in 2001 there were reports of significant liver toxicity. Over the next few years, there were more than 50 reports of kava kava-associated liver toxicity, some of which led to death or liver transplantation. Kava kava is now banned in Europe and Canada. In the United States, the FDA (Food and Drug Administration) has issued advisories about the herb. Kava kava may also cause sedation, which could worsen MS fatigue or increase the sedating effects of alcohol and some medications. Other side effects include dizziness, gastrointestinal upset, and headaches. High doses may cause skin reactions, breathing and visual difficulties, and other serious side effects. Kava kava is relatively inexpensive.

In the opinion of the Committee, kava kava may cause serious liver toxicity and other side effects. It is inexpensive and possibly effective for mild anxiety.

Padma 28

Description: Padma 28 is a complex herbal mixture that was developed by two physicians in Russia in the late 19th century.

It is composed of more than 20 different herbs. There is very limited published information about Padma 28. It is sometimes claimed to be an effective therapy for MS and several other conditions.

Rationale: Padma 28 may mildly suppress the immune system and produce antioxidant effects. Both of these actions could be therapeutic in MS.

Evaluation: Padma 28 has undergone limited study in MS. In one study of the animal model of MS, Padma 28 increased the survival time and decreased the death rate. In one published study of 100 people with MS, those who received Padma 28 treatment had a less severe clinical course than those who did not receive the herbal mixture. However, there are significant shortcomings of this study, including the lack of a placebo-treated group, the use of an unconventional neurological rating scale, and the lack of important clinical criteria for people who were in the study.

Risks/costs: Padma 28 is of low-moderate cost. There is no published information about whether long-term use is safe. In the study of people with MS, no side effects were reported.

In the opinion of the Committee, Padma 28 is of low-moderate cost and of unknown safety in MS. Although one clinical study found beneficial effects in MS, more rigorous studies are needed to determine if it is a safe or effective MS therapy.

Psyllium

Description: Psyllium is derived from the seeds of the black psyllium (*Plantago psyllium*) and blond psyllium (*Plantago ovata*) plants. It is a treatment for constipation, a condition to which some people with MS may be prone. More than four million Americans use some form of psyllium on a daily basis.

Rationale: Psyllium is a bulk-producing laxative, which means that it increases in bulk or size on exposure to water.

Evaluation: Clinical studies indicate that psyllium is an effective laxative. In the United States, the Food and Drug Administration (FDA) has approved it for use as a laxative.

Risks/costs: Psyllium is generally safe. However, if fluid intake is inadequate, psyllium may cause obstruction of the throat or intestine. Psyllium may decrease or delay the absorption of a variety of medications, including carbamazepine (Tegretol®) and warfarin (Coumadin®). To avoid this effect, oral medications should be taken 1 hour before or 4 hours after psyllium. Psyllium seeds should not be crushed because this may release chemicals that are toxic to the kidneys.

In the opinion of the Committee, psyllium is a well-tolerated and low cost herbal therapy that effectively treats constipation. Adequate fluid intake is essential to avoid obstruction of the throat or intestine.

St. John's Wort

Description: St. John's wort has been used as an antidepressant for more than 2,000 years. It is so named because it blooms around the time of the feast day of St. John the Baptist (June 24). The red pigments in its buds and flowers are associated with the blood of St. John the Baptist. Depression is a relatively common symptom in people with MS.

Rationale: In the past, it was believed that St. John's wort may produce antidepressant effects by inhibiting an enzyme known as MAO (monoamine oxidase). This does *not* appear to be the case. Rather, it may affect the brain levels of some mood-related neurochemicals, including serotonin, noradrenaline, and dopamine.

Evaluation: St. John's wort may be effective for treating mild-moderate depression. In a 1996 report, a combined analysis of

23 different clinical studies involving 1,757 people reported that St. John's wort appeared to be effective for treating mild-moderate depression. Subsequently, some studies have questioned the potency of the antidepressant effect of St. John's wort. There is no evidence that St. John's wort is effective for treating severe depression. It is unclear how the effectiveness of St. John's wort compares to that of the newer antidepressants known as selective serotonin reuptake inhibitors (SSRIs), such as fluoxetine (Prozac®), paroxetine (Paxil®), and sertraline (Zoloft®).

Risks/costs: Although St. John's wort is usually well tolerated, there are several important factors related to its use. People who are concerned they may have depression should not attempt to diagnose and treat this condition on their own. St. John's wort may produce fatigue, and consequently may worsen MS fatigue or increase the sedating effects of some medications. St. John's wort may cause a sensitivity of the skin and nerves to sunlight ("photosensitivity"), especially in those who are fair-skinned. It should be avoided by women who are pregnant or breastfeeding because of possible side effects. Finally, St. John's wort may alter the levels of multiple drugs, including anticonvulsants, antidepressants, heart medications, blood-thinning medications, and oral contraceptives. St. John's wort is inexpensive.

In the opinion of the Committee, St. John's wort is an inexpensive, generally safe herb that may be effective for treating mild-moderate depression. People with MS should not attempt to diagnose and treat their own depression. Although usually well tolerated, this herb may produce side effects and may interact with some medications.

Valerian

Description: People with MS are prone to sleep disorders. Valerian, an herb that has been used for more than 1,000 years, may be helpful for treating insomnia.

Rationale: The mechanism by which valerian might produce its actions is unclear. It may involve an effect on an anxiety- and sleep-related neurochemical known as *GABA* (gamma-aminobutyric acid).

Evaluation: Several clinical studies indicate that valerian is possibly effective for treating insomnia. Since these studies have been of variable quality, further studies are needed. Valerian is also sometimes claimed to be an effective therapy for depression, insomnia, and muscle stiffness (spasticity). However, due to limited clinical studies, its effects on these conditions are uncertain.

Risks/costs: Valerian is generally safe. It may cause sedation, which may worsen MS fatigue or increase the sedating effects of some medications. The safety of long-term use and use during pregnancy or breastfeeding has not been established. Valerian is inexpensive.

> *In the opinion of the Committee, valerian is a low-cost, generally well-tolerated therapy that may be effective for treating insomnia.*

Vitamin B_{12} (cobalamin, cyanocobalamin)

Description: Supplements of vitamin B_{12}, also known as cobalamin or cyanocobalamin, are sometimes claimed to be effective therapies for MS.

Rationale: Vitamin B_{12} is essential for maintaining normal nervous system functioning. People with vitamin B_{12} deficiency, like some people with MS, have injury to the optic nerves and the spinal cord. For these and other reasons, it is sometimes concluded that vitamin B_{12} supplements could be effective MS therapies.

Evaluation: The mechanism by which nervous system injury occurs in MS is different from that associated with vitamin B_{12} deficiency. In addition, most people with MS have normal vitamin B_{12} levels. For people who have normal vitamin B_{12} levels, there is no evidence that vitamin B_{12} supplements provide any definite beneficial effects. Importantly, there is a small subgroup of people with MS who have vitamin B_{12} deficiency. In that case, treatment with vitamin B_{12} is recommended. One study of six people with progressive MS found that massive doses of vitamin B_{12} did not provide any definite clinical benefit over a 6-month period. In another study, 138 people with MS were placed in two treatment groups, one of which was treated with vitamin B_{12} alone and the other with the "Cari Loder regime" (vitamin B_{12} along with two other compounds, phenylalanine and lofepramine). In this 24-week study, both groups showed mild neurological improvement after 2 weeks of treatment. The group treated with the "Cari Loder regime" showed some additional mild neurological improvement and had mild relief of some MS symptoms, including fatigue. The significance of the small therapeutic effects seen in this study is not clear. Further studies of this treatment regimen are needed.

Risks/costs: Vitamin B_{12} supplements are usually well tolerated. Rarely, vitamin B_{12} may cause diarrhea, rashes, and itching. Vitamin B_{12} is inexpensive.

In the opinion of the Committee, vitamin B_{12} supplements are inexpensive and generally safe. For people with MS who have normal vitamin B_{12} levels, supplements of vitamin B_{12} do not provide any definite benefit. For people with MS who have low vitamin B_{12} levels, vitamin B_{12} supplements are recommended. One study with vitamin B_{12}, phenylalanine, and lofepramine has shown mild beneficial effects; further studies of this therapy are needed.

Vitamin D and Calcium

Description: Vitamin D and calcium have multiple actions in the body, including an important role in maintaining bone density. Vitamin D and calcium are relevant to people with MS for two reasons. First, people with MS are at risk for developing osteoporosis and a less severe form of decreased bone density known as osteopenia. In addition, vitamin D and calcium have effects on immune system function.

Rationale: People with MS are prone to decreased bone density, and vitamin D and calcium are important in maintaining bone density. In addition, vitamin D mildly suppresses immune system function in a way that could be therapeutic for people with MS.

Evaluation: A possible therapeutic effect for vitamin D in MS is suggested by several studies. In the animal model of MS, disease severity is worsened by vitamin D deficiency and improved by vitamin D supplementation. Epidemiologic studies indicate that the use of vitamin D supplements is associated with a decreased risk of developing MS. Unfortunately, there is very limited clinical trial information about vitamin D and MS. A preliminary report of a small, short-term study of 11 people with MS found that treatment with 19-nor, a form of vitamin D, did not produce significant benefits on the basis of clinical tests and magnetic resonance imaging (MRI) measures.

Risks/costs: In reasonable doses, vitamin D and calcium are usually well tolerated. Calcium may interfere with the absorption of some medications (antibiotics, thyroid medication, osteoporosis medication) and minerals (iron, magnesium, zinc). In high doses, vitamin D and calcium may cause multiple side effects. Vitamin D and calcium are inexpensive.

In the opinion of the Committee, vitamin D and calcium are low-cost, generally safe therapies. Treatment with these supplements should be considered in people who are at risk for low bone density or have known decreased bone density. There are suggestive studies that vitamin D and calcium could have a therapeutic effect on the disease course in MS, but additional studies are needed to determine if there is any definite effect.

Zinc

Description: Zinc is a mineral that plays an important role in many biological processes, including the functioning of the immune system and the synthesis and breakdown of essential molecules in the body. It is sometimes recommended as a therapy for MS. In the 1880s, zinc phosphate, a form of zinc, was actually used as a treatment for MS.

Rationale: The reason that zinc is recommended for MS is not always clear. Sometimes it is recommended because it is involved in the biochemical pathway of the polyunsaturated fatty acids (see below under "Diets"). In addition, zinc has effects on immune system function.

Evaluation: There are no well-designed clinical studies that have evaluated the effects of zinc supplementation on MS. Although polyunsaturated fatty acids may have a therapeutic effect in MS, it is not clear that zinc supplements taken along with polyunsaturated fatty acids provide any additional therapeutic effect. Zinc has multiple effects on the immune system, including the activation of immune cells known as T cells. Zinc supplements may cause worsening in the animal model of MS. There are reports of people with high blood levels of zinc (and low blood levels of copper) who develop an MS-like condition ("copper-deficiency myelopathy"), and limited studies indicate a possible increased risk of MS in people exposed to high environmental levels of zinc.

Risks/costs: Due to the immune-stimulating effect of zinc and the possible association of high zinc levels with an MS-like condition, zinc supplements pose theoretical risks in people with MS. Chronic use of high doses may cause copper deficiency, which may produce neurological symptoms that are similar to those of MS. Chronic, high dose zinc may also impair immune function and adversely affect cholesterol levels. Zinc supplements are inexpensive.

In the opinion of the Committee, zinc is a low-cost therapy with theoretical risks and no known beneficial effect in MS. High doses of zinc may produce multiple side effects, including neurological symptoms that may be similar to those of MS.

Diets

Many diets have been proposed as effective MS therapies. For many of these diets, there is no clear underlying rationale or clinical evidence to support their use in MS. Diets for MS that are *not* supported by a strong rationale or clinical data include allergen-free diets, gluten-free diets, pectin- and fructose-restricted diets, severely sugar-restricted diets, and diets that reduce or eliminate processed foods.

On the basis of scientific, epidemiological, animal model, and clinical trial studies, there is suggestive evidence that diets that are low in saturated fats and high in polyunsaturated fatty acids (PUFAs) may have a therapeutic effect in MS. PUFAs include omega-3 and omega-6 fatty acids. Omega-6 fatty acids include compounds known as linoleic acid and gamma-linolenic acid. Examples of omega-3 fatty acids include eicosapentanoic acid (EPA), docosahexanoic acid (DHA), and alpha-linolenic acid (ALA). The remainder of this section will review three PUFA-related dietary approaches. The first PUFA-enriched diet that was extensively studied in MS was the Swank diet. Subsequently, several MS clinical studies evaluated the effects of supplementation with omega-6 and omega-3 fatty acids.

The Swank Diet

Description: In the 1940s, Dr. Roy Swank developed a dietary approach that has been reported to be an effective treatment for MS. With this diet, saturated fat intake is decreased to 15 grams or less daily, high-fat dairy products are excluded, frequent fish meals are recommended, and 10–15 grams of fluid vegetable oil and 5 grams of cod-liver oil are added to the daily diet.

Rationale: This diet was developed due to the apparent association of dietary fat intake with MS. Specifically, early epidemiological studies indicated that MS is less common in populations that consume relatively low levels of saturated fats and relatively high levels of polyunsaturated fatty acids (PUFAs). Studies conducted subsequent to the development of the Swank diet have provided additional rationale for this type of dietary approach (see below under "Supplementation with Omega-6 Fatty Acids" and "Supplementation with Omega-3 Fatty Acids").

Evaluation: There have been several reports of the initial group of people with MS who were treated with the Swank diet. In one of these reports, 134 people with MS were monitored for 34 years on the Swank diet. In the first year on the diet, the rate of MS attacks was decreased by 70 percent relative to the attack rate prior to entering the study. Unfortunately, there was no placebo-treated group in this study. As a result, the people in the study were compared to people with MS reported in the medical literature who did not receive any type of MS treatment ("natural history controls"). When this type of comparison was done, it was found that people on the diet had less frequent attacks, less progression of neurological disability, and decreased mortality. These beneficial effects were greatest in those who adhered strictly to the diet and those who were mildly affected or were early in the course of the disease. Although these findings are encouraging, this study has significant shortcomings. As noted, there was no placebo-treated group. In addition, people who were treated were not randomly selected for treatment ("randomized") and the examining clinicians and the treated patients were not "blind" to whether they were being treated. Due to these and other shortcomings, this study is not rigorous enough to provide definitive conclusions about the effectiveness of this dietary approach.

Risks/costs: This diet is usually well tolerated. Long-term adherence to the diet may not be possible because the recommended food is not appealing. Due to the decreased meat intake in the

Swank diet, people who use this dietary approach should be certain that protein intake is adequate. Although cod-liver oil, one component of this diet, is generally safe, it may rarely cause adverse effects. Cod-liver oil may have a blood-thinning effect and should be used with caution by those who take aspirin or anticoagulant medication, are undergoing surgery, or have bleeding disorders. Diabetics should also use cod-liver oil with caution. Finally, cod-liver oil contains relatively high concentrations of vitamin A, which may be toxic in doses greater than 10,000 IU. The Swank diet is inexpensive.

> *In the opinion of the Committee, the Swank diet is an inexpensive and relatively safe dietary approach that has produced suggestive results in a limited MS clinical study. Due to the inadequacies of the Swank diet clinical trial, definitive conclusions cannot be made about the safety or effectiveness of this diet in people with MS. Further study of the Swank diet is needed. The safety and effectiveness of the Swank diet in combination with disease-modifying medications (interferons, glatiramer acetate, mitoxantrone, and natalizumab) has not been studied.*

Supplementation with Omega-6 Fatty Acids

Description: Supplementation with omega-6 fatty acids is an approach that increases the intake of polyunsaturated fatty acids (PUFAs). Most studies of omega-6 fatty acid supplementation have used sunflower seed oil or evening primrose oil. Other dietary supplements that contain omega-6 fatty acids include flaxseed oil, borage seed oil, black currant seed oil, and spirulina (blue-green algae).

Rationale: As noted for the Swank diet (see above), epidemiological studies indicate that a high intake of PUFAs may be associated with a lower risk of developing MS. There are other findings that support the use of a diet enriched in omega-6 fatty acids. Some, but not all, studies have shown that the blood levels of PUFAs are decreased in people with MS. In addition, scientific studies show that in the body PUFAs are converted to compounds known as leukotrienes and prostaglandins. These compounds have antiinflammatory effects and immune system-modulating effects that, on a theoretical basis, could be therapeutic for MS.

Evaluation: In the animal model of MS, disease severity is worsened by deficiencies in omega-6 fatty acids and lessened by supplementation with omega-6 fatty acids. In people with RRMS, three placebo-controlled clinical trials have evaluated supplementation with omega-6 fatty acids. In these studies, the treated group received sunflower seed oil, which contains an omega-6 fatty acid known as linoleic acid. In two of these studies, there was a significant decrease in the duration and severity of MS attacks. In the other study, there was not a therapeutic effect. A re-analysis of these three studies, for which not all of the original data was available, showed that people with mild disability had a statistically significant decrease in progression of disability and a statistically significant decrease in attack severity and duration; people with moderate-severe disability had no significant change in disability and a statistically significant decrease in attack severity and duration. In studies of people with progressive MS, omega-6 fatty acid supplementation has not been effective. Evening primrose oil, a dietary supplement that contains an omega-6 fatty acid known as gamma-linolenic acid, has not produced therapeutic effects in people with relapsing-remitting or progressive disease.

Risks/costs: Supplementation with omega-6 fatty acids is usually well tolerated. The safety of long-term supplementation with omega-6 fatty acids has not been well studied. A concern has been raised that linoleic acid supplementation may increase the risk of some forms of cancer, but this has not been proven. Since supplementation with PUFAs may cause vitamin E deficiency, supplementation with vitamin E may be necessary. Evening primrose oil, and perhaps other gamma-linolenic acid-containing supplements (black currant seed oil, borage seed oil, spirulina), may rarely provoke seizures. Also, gamma-linolenic acid-containing supplements may have blood-thinning effects. Omega-6 fatty acid supplements may increase triglyceride levels and thus should be used with caution by people with elevated triglycerides. One specific supplement, borage seed oil, may contain liver toxins known as pyrrolizidine alkaloids. The safety of black currant seed oil has not been well studied. Spirulina products may contain heavy metals, bacteria, and other contaminants. The safety of omega-6 fatty acid supplementation in women who are pregnant or breastfeeding is not known. Supplementation with omega-6 fatty acids is inexpensive.

In the opinion of the Committee, omega-6 fatty acid supplementation is an inexpensive and generally well-tolerated approach that has produced suggestive therapeutic effects in trials with relapsing-remitting MS. Further studies are needed to determine if it is definitely effective. The safety and effectiveness of this approach in combination with disease-modifying medications (interferons, glatiramer acetate, mitoxantrone, and natalizumab) are not known.

Supplementation with Omega-3 Fatty Acids

Description: This approach increases the intake of omega-3 fatty acids, which include eicosapentanoic acid (EPA), docosahexanoic acid (DHA), and alpha-linolenic acid (ALA). EPA and DHA are present in relatively high levels in fish, especially fatty fish such as salmon, Atlantic herring, Atlantic mackerel, bluefin tuna, and sardines. Dietary supplements containing EPA and DHA include fish oil and cod-liver oil. Rich sources of ALA include flaxseed oil, canola oil, and walnut oil.

Rationale: The rationale for this approach is similar to that outlined for the Swank diet and supplementation with omega-6 fatty acids (see above, under "Swank Diet" and "Supplementa-

tion with Omega-6 Fatty Acids"). In addition, immunologic studies indicate that, among the polyunsaturated fatty acids (PUFAs),
the omega-3 fatty acids exert the most potent antiinflammatory
and immune-modulating effects. Also, omega-3 fatty acids appear to be important in forming and maintaining myelin, a part
of the nervous system that is injured in MS.

Evaluation: Studies of omega-3 fatty acid supplementation in
the animal model of MS are limited and conflicting. The most
rigorous clinical study of this approach was a placebo-controlled
trial of fish oil in people with RRMS. There was a trend for the
treated group to show less disease progression, fewer attacks,
and decreased attack duration, but these findings were not statistically significant. Therapeutic effects were noted in two uncontrolled studies, one with cod-liver oil, calcium, and magnesium,
and the other with fish oil, other dietary supplements, and dietary
advice. A small study evaluated omega-3 fatty acid supplementation in combination with interferons or glatiramer acetate. People
were treated with their MS medications along with either fish
oil and a very low-fat diet or with olive oil and a low-fat diet.
There was a trend for improved physical and emotional functioning in those taking fish oil. Both dietary interventions were
associated with a decrease in relapse rate.

Risks/costs: Supplementation with modest doses of fish oil is
generally safe. In the United States, the Food and Drug Administration (FDA) has classified fish oils as "generally regarded as
safe." A 7-year study of fish oil use in nearly 300 people did
not find any serious side effects. The long-term safety of other
omega-3 fatty acid supplements is not known. Increased dietary
intake of ALA may increase the risk of prostate cancer. Although
fish oil supplements generally do not have a significant amount
of mercury, some fish, such as shark, swordfish, and king mackerel, do contain relatively high mercury levels. Fish and flaxseed
oil may have a blood-thinning effect. Fish oil may impair lung
function in those who are aspirin-sensitive. High doses of fish
oil may increase blood sugar levels in diabetics. High doses of

flaxseed oil may produce cyanide toxicity. There are potential side effects that are specifically associated with cod-liver oil (see above, under "Swank diet"). For women who are pregnant or breastfeeding, the safety of omega-3 fatty acid supplements, including fish oil, is not known. Supplementation with omega-3 fatty acids is inexpensive.

In the opinion of the Committee, omega-3 fatty acid supplementation is inexpensive and generally well tolerated. In limited MS studies, this approach has produced suggestive, but not definitive, therapeutic effects. A preliminary report indicates a possible beneficial effect of fish oil supplements in combination with interferons or glatiramer acetate. Further study of omega-3 fatty acid supplementation is needed to determine whether it is definitely effective in MS and whether it is safe and effective in combination with disease-modifying medications.

Feldenkrais

Description: Feldenkrais, a type of bodywork, teaches comfortable and efficient body movements. It is claimed to improve multiple symptoms and to provide therapeutic effects for people with MS. People with disabilities can do Feldenkrais. There are two types of Feldenkrais. With the Awareness Through Movement (ATM) method, the focus is on the motion of the body during simple movements such as bending or walking. The other technique, Functional Integration (FI), involves an instructor who actually manipulates muscles and joints during movement.

Rationale: The retraining of movements with Feldenkrais is believed to increase the efficiency and comfort of body movements. This is claimed to improve walking stability, increase strength and coordination, and decrease stress.

Evaluation: Feldenkrais has undergone very limited investigation in MS and other conditions. In one small study, 20 people with MS were treated for 8 weeks with either Feldenkrais or "sham" sessions. The treated group had significantly decreased stress and a trend for decreased anxiety relative to the "sham" group. There were no significant effects on arm function, overall level of function, and multiple other MS symptoms. This study was not rigorous enough to be conclusive. Additional study with more people with MS, longer treatment times, and more rigorous study design are needed.

Risks/costs: Feldenkrais is generally safe. ATM classes are low cost. FI sessions are moderate cost.

In the opinion of the Committee, Feldenkrais is a low-moderate cost, generally well tolerated therapy that has produced decreased stress in one small study in MS. Further studies are needed to determine whether Feldenkrais has any definite therapeutic effects in MS.

Guided Imagery and Relaxation

Description: Guided imagery, also known as *imagery* or *visualization*, is a relaxation method. It is often used in combination with other relaxation methods, such as progressive muscle relaxation. It is claimed to be effective for treating a variety of symptoms that may occur in people with MS, including anxiety, depression, and pain. In guided imagery, an individual creates mental images that have specific effects on the body and mind.

Rationale: It is believed that the mental processes involved in guided imagery induce relaxation or other bodily changes that have therapeutic effects.

Evaluation: In one published study of 33 people with MS, it was found that anxiety was decreased in those who used guided imagery and relaxation. These methods had no effect on depression or many other MS symptoms. In studies of other conditions, imagery and other relaxation methods were found to be possibly effective for treating anxiety, depression, pain, and insomnia.

Larger and more rigorous studies of guided imagery and other relaxation methods are needed.

Risks/costs: Guided imagery and relaxation are usually well tolerated. Relaxation may cause or worsen muscle stiffness. Imagery may cause fear of losing control, anxiety, and disturbing thoughts. As a result, people with psychiatric conditions should use it with caution. Guided imagery is inexpensive.

In the opinion of the Committee, guided imagery and relaxation are generally well-tolerated and inexpensive therapies that may decrease anxiety and other symptoms. Further studies are needed to determine whether these therapies are definitely effective for anxiety or other MS-related symptoms.

Hyperbaric Oxygen

Description: Hyperbaric oxygen (HBO) treatment is a form of oxygen therapy in which a person breathes oxygen under increased pressure in a specially designed chamber. It is claimed that HBO is effective for MS and many other diseases.

Rationale: The oxygen content of the blood increases with the use of HBO. This results in an increased amount of oxygen in different body tissues. It is believed that the increased oxygen levels in the blood and tissues are therapeutic for a variety of medical conditions.

Evaluation: HBO is an accepted treatment for a limited number of specific medical conditions, including burns, severe infections, decompression sickness (due to deep-sea diving), radiation-induced tissue injury, and carbon monoxide poisoning. Unfortunately, there is no strong evidence to support the use of HBO in MS and many other diseases. There are no clear theoretical reasons as to why increased oxygen levels would be therapeutic in MS. The human clinical studies of HBO in MS can be confusing. This is because an early study of HBO in MS, reported in 1983, found that it was effective. This study was published in a prestigious medical journal, *The New England Journal of Medicine*. This single study is still sometimes provided as evidence for the effectiveness of HBO for MS. However, subsequent to the 1983 study, many clinical trials were conducted and generally found that HBO did not produce beneficial effects in people with MS. A mild improvement in bladder function was reported in a few studies. Large independent reviews of all of the published HBO and MS clinical trials were published in 1995 and 2004. Both reviews conclude that there is no consistent therapeutic effect of HBO in people with MS and that HBO should not be used to treat MS. In addition, the 2004 article, a *Cochrane Database Review*, concludes that, on the basis of existing evidence, further studies of HBO in MS are not justified.

Risks/costs: HBO is usually well tolerated. Reversible, mild visual symptoms may occur. Rarely, HBO may cause serious side effects, including seizures, collapsed lungs, pressure injury to the ear, and cataracts. HBO is expensive.

In the opinion of the Committee, HBO is an expensive therapy with rare, but serious, side effects that, on the basis of multiple clinical trials, does not produce any consistent therapeutic effects in people with MS.

Magnetic Field Therapy (Electromagnetic Therapy)

Description: There are two main forms of unconventional therapy with electromagnetic fields: static, permanent magnets and pulsed electromagnetic fields. Static magnetic therapy involves the use of magnetized devices such as bracelets, belts, and mattress pads. Pulsed electromagnetic field therapy, which has been more extensively studied in MS than static magnets, uses devices that produce pulsing, electromagnetic fields at a specific frequency. In one MS study, devices with a strong, pulsing magnetic field were placed on the spine. In other studies, small devices with weak, pulsing magnetic fields were placed on the legs or specific acupuncture points.

Rationale: Multiple mechanisms have been proposed to explain possible therapeutic effects of magnetic fields in MS and other conditions. With strong magnets placed on the spine, it has been proposed that the magnetic field activates nerves in the spinal cord in such a way that there is a decreased tendency towards spasticity. For weaker magnetic fields, it is generally claimed that there are disease-associated electrical imbalances and that these can be corrected with magnetic therapy. It is believed that devices placed on acupuncture points may have acupuncture-like effects, such as altering the release of pain-relieving chemicals (opioids) in the body. Other effects have also been proposed, including activation of the sympathetic skin response, alteration of the flow of electrically charged atoms (such as calcium) through channels in the membranes of different cells in the body, alteration of the levels of a hormone, melatonin, and modulation of immune system cells.

Evaluation: There have been four placebo-controlled clinical trials of pulsed electromagnetic therapy in MS. Three of these have involved weak magnetic fields; one involved strong magnetic fields applied to the spine. In these studies, the effect of therapy on various MS symptoms was assessed. In the study of strong magnetic fields applied to the spine, spasticity was specifically evaluated and was found to be significantly decreased in the treated group compared to the placebo group. In the three studies with the weaker devices, beneficial effects on spasticity were found in some but not all studies. Similarly, in some but not necessarily all studies, improvement was noted in other MS symptoms, including pain, bladder function, hand function, fatigue, and quality of life. Given the variable findings and lack of rigor in some of these studies, further investigation is needed to clarify whether this therapy has definite beneficial effects. In addition to these clinical trials involving groups of people with MS, there are case reports in which magnetic therapy has improved various MS symptoms in individuals with MS. It is difficult to make conclusions from these studies because each report involves only a single person.

Risks/costs: Short-term use of magnetic field therapy is usually well tolerated. The long-term effects of this treatment have not been investigated. Treatment with a strong magnet on the spine may produce dizziness and a band-like sensation around the torso. The weaker devices may cause headaches. Pregnant women and people with pacemakers or other electronic medical devices should consult with their physician before using these devices. Devices with a weak magnetic field are of low-moderate cost. Devices with a strong magnetic field are for experimental use and are not generally available.

In the opinion of the Committee, pulsed electromagnetic field therapy is a low-moderate cost, generally well-tolerated therapy. Several MS clinical trials of variable quality have produced suggestive results, especially for spasticity. Further studies are needed to determine if this therapy has definite therapeutic effects in MS.

Massage

Description: Massage, one of the oldest forms of treatment, is a form of bodywork in which soft tissue is manipulated with pressure and traction. The common forms of massage in Western countries are derived from Swedish massage, which was developed by a Swedish physician in the nineteenth century.

Rationale: There are various explanations for the possible therapeutic effects of massage. It is believed that massage improves the circulation of blood and lymph and thereby improves the delivery of oxygen and the removal of allegedly harmful toxins from tissues. Massage is also claimed to decrease muscle stiffness and to release "endorphins," pain-relieving chemicals. Finally, the simple act of touching, which is *not* the focus of conventional medical treatment, is claimed to convey feelings of comfort, caring, and acceptance.

Evaluation: There is one study of massage therapy in people with MS. In this 5-week study, 24 people with MS were assigned either to a control group that received "standard medical care" or to a massage treatment group that received standard medical care in combination with twice-weekly, in-home massage therapy. Importantly, the control group did not receive any type of "placebo" therapy. Also, at the start of the study, the control and treatment groups were significantly different with regard to level of disability. Relative to the start of the study, the treatment group exhibited less anxiety and depression after the first massage session and improvement in self-esteem, body image, "image of disease progression," and social functioning at the end of the 5-week study. In the statistical analysis, comparisons were generally made within the treatment group. The results of this study are promising but not definitive. Larger studies with more well-matched groups and more rigorous study design are needed.

Risks/costs: Massage is usually well tolerated. Minor side effects include headache, lethargy, and muscle pain. More serious side effects, such as bone fractures and bleeding into the liver, are possible but rare. Massage should be avoided or used with caution by people with the following conditions: clotted blood vessels (thrombosis), burns, skin infections, open wounds, bone fractures, osteoporosis, cancer, pregnancy, and heart disease. The cost of massage depends on the frequency and duration of treatment. It is of low-moderate cost.

In the opinion of the Committee, massage is a low-moderate cost, generally safe therapy that has produced promising results in one small MS study. Further studies are needed to determine whether massage is definitely effective for treating MS symptoms.

Neural Therapy

Description: Neural therapy is a type of energy therapy that was developed in Europe in the 1920s. It involves injecting small quantities of local anesthetic under the skin in specific locations, which may be acupuncture points or old scars.

Rationale: Neural therapy is believed to supply energy to injured tissues or to remove blockages in the flow of energy. In people with MS, it is claimed that this therapy may restore normal conduction to *demyelinated* nerves, which are nerves that have MS-induced injury to their insulating layer. It is not clear how injections under the skin could quickly improve the function of demyelinated nerves in the brain and spinal cord.

Evaluation: There is one study of neural therapy in MS. This two-part investigation involved injections in the ankles and head. In one part of the study, which did not involve a control group, 40 people with MS were treated in a variable way that was dependent on their clinical course. It was found that some type of objective improvement occurred in 65 percent of people. The improvement usually occurred within minutes of the first series of injections. In the second phase of the study, 21 people with MS received active or placebo (saline injections) treatment for 1 week, and then all of the participants received active treatment for 1 week. At the end of the first week, the group that received active treatment showed more improvement than the placebo group. At the end of the second week, 76 percent of all participants showed some type of improvement. This study provides suggestive results, but longer term, larger, and more rigorous studies are needed.

Risks/costs: There is limited information about the safety of neural therapy. It is believed to be generally safe. Repeated injections on a long-term basis may cause scarring. Allergies to the local anesthetic may occur. In the MS study, it was noted that worsening might occur if injections are given during a time when there is improvement. The cost of neural therapy depends on the duration of treatment. A brief course of therapy is inexpensive.

In the opinion of the Committee, neural therapy is an inexpensive and generally safe therapy that has pro-

duced suggestive results in one study. The underlying rationale for this therapy is not clear. To clarify whether neural therapy has any definite therapeutic effects in MS, further studies are needed.

Reflexology

Description: Reflexology is a type of bodywork in which manual pressure is applied to specific areas. These areas, which are usually on the feet but may also be on the hands and ears, are thought to correspond to specific parts of the body.

Rationale: It is believed that pressure at specific reflexology sites improves energy flow to the corresponding body parts. This improved energy flow is claimed to improve health.

Evaluation: In one controlled study of reflexology, 71 people with MS were treated for 11 weeks with either reflexology or nonspecific massage of the calf area. There was a relatively high dropout rat in this short study, and only 53 people completed the study. Relative to the control group, the people treated with reflexology exhibited significant improvement in paresthesias, urinary symptoms, and spasticity. To determine if reflexology has definite therapeutic effects in MS, larger and more rigorous studies with lower dropout rates are needed.

Risks/costs: Reflexology is generally well tolerated. Mild side effects include fatigue, foot pain, and changes in bowel and bladder function. Reflexology should be avoided or used with caution by people with bone or joint conditions of the feet, and by those with other foot conditions such as gout, ulcers, and vascular disease.

In the opinion of the Committee, reflexology is a low-moderate cost, low-risk therapy that has produced promising results in MS in one study. More rigorous investigation is needed to determine if reflexology has definite therapeutic effects in MS.

Tai Chi

Description: Tai chi is a traditional Chinese martial art that has been practiced for centuries in China. There has been recent interest in tai chi in some Western countries. Tai chi is characterized by a series of body postures that are linked by slow, graceful movements. Tai chi may be modified for people with disabilities.

Rationale: Tai chi may be interpreted from a traditional Chinese or Western perspective. According to ancient Chinese philosophy, there are two opposing life forces, yin and yang. Tai chi is believed to be a way to stabilize these energies and create emotional balance. From a Western scientific perspective, tai chi may be viewed as a form of physical exercise that may produce beneficial neurological and cardiovascular effects. Specifically, tai chi may improve cardiovascular function and increase strength, coordination, and balance in a way similar to exercise.

Evaluation: In one study of tai chi in MS, 19 people with MS with variable levels of disability were enrolled in an 8-week tai chi program. At the end of the program, there was improvement in walking speed and muscle stiffness. There was also improvement in vitality, social and emotional functioning, and ability to carry out physical and emotional roles. Significant limitations of this study are that it was relatively small, there was no placebo-treated group, and non-standard measures and non-blinded assessment were used. Another study of 16 people with MS used the tai chi principle of "mindfulness of movement," which involves developing moment-to-moment awareness of movement, breathing, and posture. Relative to the control group, which received "current available care," the treated group did not improve in balance but did improve in multiple MS-associated symptoms, as assessed by patients and by their relatives. Relative to pretreatment, the treated group improved in balance. This study had a relatively large drop-out rate, involved a small number of people, and did not use objective and "blinded" clinicians for assessment. Larger and more rigorous studies are needed to determine if tai chi is definitely effective for treating MS-related symptoms.

Risks/costs: Tai chi is usually well tolerated. Mild side effects include strained muscles and joints. It may worsen MS-related fatigue. There is a report of tai chi worsening electrical sensations in the arms and back (Lhermitte's phenomena) in an individual with MS. It should be avoided or used with caution by those with severe osteoporosis, acute low back pain, significant joint injuries, and bone fractures. Tai chi is low-moderate cost.

In the opinion of the Committee, tai chi is a low-moderate cost, generally well-tolerated therapy that has produced improvement in multiple symptoms in one small MS study. Larger and more rigorous studies are needed.

Yoga

Description: Yoga is a mind-body approach that was developed in India thousands of years ago. Yoga, which is derived from the Sanskrit word for *union*, is meant to unite the mind, body, and spirit. In *hatha yoga,* one of the more popular forms of yoga, the three main components are breathing, meditation, and posture. Yoga may be modified for people with disabilities.

Rationale: According to traditional Indian teaching, yoga increases the body's stores of vital energy, known as *prana*, and facilitates the flow of energy. From a Western perspective, yoga may be viewed as a multifaceted approach that may potentially produce emotional benefits resulting from relaxation, and physical benefits, such as increased strength and decreased muscle stiffness, as a result of performing the yoga postures.

Evaluation: In spite of yoga's popularity in some countries, there are very limited clinical studies of its effects in MS and other diseases. There is one well-designed, controlled trial of yoga in MS. In this 6-month study, 69 people with MS were randomized to a control group that received no intervention, or to groups that were treated with conventional exercise or yoga. Relative to the control group, the yoga and conventional exercise groups had significant decreases in fatigue on the basis of two different measures. There were no consistent effects of yoga or conventional exercise on cognitive function or mood. It is not possible to determine whether yoga's effects on fatigue were to the result of the yoga itself or resulted from other factors, such as a placebo response or benefits from being in a social setting.

Risks/costs: Yoga is generally safe. In the clinical trial of yoga and MS, it was not associated with any serious adverse effects. Difficult postures or vigorous exercise should be avoided or done with caution by pregnant women, people with significant heart, lung, or bone conditions, or people with heat sensitivity, fatigue, and decreased balance. Yoga is a low-cost therapy, especially when it is done in groups.

In the opinion of the Committee, yoga is a low-cost, generally well-tolerated therapy that may decrease fatigue. Additional studies of yoga in MS are needed.

Guide to Further Reading

Unconventional Medicine: Generally

- Barnes PM, Powell-Griner E, McFann K, et al. Complementary and alternative medicine use among adults: United States, 2002. *Advance Data* 2004; 343:1–19.

- Bowling AC. *Alternative Medicine and Multiple Sclerosis.* New York: Demos Medical Publishing, 2001.

- Eisenberg D, Davis R, Ettner S, et al. Trends in alternative medicine use in the United States, 1990–1997. *JAMA* 1998; 280:1569–75.

- Marrie R, Hadjimichael O, Vollmer T. Predictors of alternative medicine use by multiple sclerosis patients. *Mult Scler* 2003; 9:461–466.

- Stuifbergen AK, Harrison TC. Complementary and alternative therapy use in persons with multiple sclerosis. *Rehab Nurs* 2003; 28:141–147.

Acupuncture and Traditional Chinese Medicine

- Bowling AC. *Alternative Medicine and Multiple Sclerosis*. New York: Demos Medical Publishing, 2001:27–35.

- NIH Consensus Development Panel on Acupuncture. *JAMA* 1998; 280:1518–24.

- Smith MO, Rabinowitz N. Acupuncture treatment of multiple sclerosis: Two detailed clinical presentations. *Amer J Acupuncture* 1986; 14:143–6.

- Spoerel WE, Paty DW, Kertesz A, et al. Acupuncture and multiple sclerosis. *CMA Journal* 1974; 110:751.

- Wang Y, Hashimoto S, Ramsum D, et al. A pilot study of the use of alternative medicine in multiple sclerosis patients with special focus on acupuncture. *Neurology* 1999; 52:A550.

Bee Venom Therapy

- Bowling AC. *Alternative Medicine and Multiple Sclerosis*. New York: Demos Medical Publishing, 2001:46–51.

- Lublin FD, Oshinsky RJ, Perreault, M, et al. Effect of honey bee venom on EAE. *Neurol* 1998; 50:A424.

- Nam KW, Je KH, Lee JH, et al. Inhibition of COX-2 activity and proinflammatory cytokines (TNF-alpha and IL-1 beta) production by water-soluble sub-fractionated parts from bee (Apis mellifera) venom. *Arch Pharm Res* 2003; 26:383–388.

- Song H-S, Wray SH. Bee sting optic neuritis. *J Clin Neuro-Ophthalmol* 1991; 11:45–49.

Cannabis (Marijuana)

- Baker D, Pryce G, Giovannoni G, et al. The therapeutic potential of cannabis. *Lancet Neurol* 2003; 2:291–298.

- Bowling AC. Worthless weed or pot of gold? *Int J MS Care* 2004; 5:138,166.

- Clark AJ, Ware MA, Yazer E, et al. Patterns of cannabis use among patients with multiple sclerosis. *Neurol* 2004; 62:2098–2100.

- Killestein J, Hoogervorst ELJ, Reif M, et al. Immunomodulatory effects of orally administered cannabinoids in multiple sclerosis. *J Neuroimmunol* 2003; 137:140–143.

- Zajicek J, Fox P, Sanders H, et al. Cannabinoids for treatment of spasticity and other symptoms related to multiple sclerosis (CAMS study): Multicentre randomized placebo-controlled trial. *Lancet* 2003; 362: 1517–1526.

- Zajicek J, Sanders HP, Wright DE, et al. Cannabinoids in multiple sclerosis (CAMS) study: safety and efficacy data for 52 weeks follow-up. *J Neurol Neurosurg Psych* 2005; in press.

Chiropractic Medicine

- Bowling AC. *Alternative Medicine and Multiple Sclerosis.* New York: Demos Medical Publishing, 2001:59–62.

- Elster E. Eighty-one patients with multiple sclerosis and Parkinson's disease undergoing upper cervical chiropractic care to correct vertebral subluxation: A retrospective analysis. *J Vertebral Sublux Res* Aug. 4, 2004:1–9.

- Ernst E, Harkness E. Spinal manipulation: A systematic review of sham-controlled, double-blind, randomized clinical trials. *J Pain Symptom Manage* 2001; 2:879–889.

- Ferreira ML, Ferreira PH, Latimer J, et al. Efficacy of spinal manipulative therapy for low back pain of less than three months' duration. *J Manipul Physiol Ther* 2003; 26:593–601.

- Kaptchuk TJ, Eisenberg DM. Chiropractic-origins, controversies, and contributions. *Arch Intern Med* 1998; 158:2215–24.

- Smith WS, Johnston SC, Skalabrin EJ, et al. Spinal manipulative therapy is an independent risk factor for vertebral artery dissection. *Neurol* 2003; 60:1424–1428.

Cooling Therapy

- Capell E, Gardella M, Leandri M, et al. Lowering body temperature with a cooling suit as symptomatic treatment for thermosensitve multiple sclerosis patients. *Ital J Neurol Scis* 1995; 16:533–9.

- Flensner G, Lindencrona C. The cooling-suit: A study of ten multiple sclerosis patients' experience in daily life. *J Adv Nursing* 1999; 29:1444–53.

- Guthrie TC, Nelson DA. Influence of temperature changes on multiple sclerosis: Critical review of mechanisms and research potential. *J Neurol Scis* 1995; 129:1–8.

- Ku YT, Montgomery LD, Wenzel KC, et al. Physiologic and thermal responses of male and female patients with multiple sclerosis to head and neck cooling. *Am J Phys Medicine & Rehab* 1999; 78:447–56.

- Schwid SR, Petrie MD, Murray R, et al.; NASA/MS Cooling Study Group. A randomized controlled study of the acute and chronic effects of cooling therapy for MS. *Neurol* 2003; 60:1955–1960.

Dental Amalgam Removal

- Bates MN, Fawcett J, Garrett N, et al. Health effects of dental amalgam exposure: A retrospective cohort study. *Int J Epid* 2004; 33:1–9.

- Casetta I, Invernizzi M, Granieri E. Multiple sclerosis and dental amalgam: Case-control study in Ferrara, Italy. *Neuroepid* 2001; 20:134–137.

- Ekstrand J, Bjorkman L, Edlund C, et al. Toxicological aspects on the release and systemic uptake of mercury from dental amalgam. *Eur J Oral Scis* 1998; 106:678–86.

- Eley BM, Cox SW. The release, absorption, and possible health effects of mercury from dental amalgam: A review of recent findings. *Brit Dental J* 1993; 175:355–362.

- NIH Conference Assessment. Effects and side-effects of dental restorative materials. *Adv Dental Res* 1992; 6:1–144.

Dietary Supplements: Antioxidants

- Bowling AC. *Alternative Medicine: And Multiple Sclerosis.* New York: Demos Medical Publishing, 2001: 198–199.

- Bowling AC, Stewart TM. Current complementary and alternative therapies for multiple sclerosis. *Curr Treat Options Neurol* 2003; 5:55–68.

- Mai J, Sorenson P, Hansen J. High dose antioxidant supplementation to MS patients: Effects on glutathione peroxidase, clinical safety, and absorption of selenium. *Biol Trace Elem Res* 1990; 24:109–117.

- Marcucci GH, Jones RE, McKeon GP, et al. Alpha lipoic acid inhibits T cell migration into the spinal cord and suppresses and treats experimental autoimmune encephalomyelitis. *J Neuroimmunol* 2002; 131:104–114.

- Scott GS, Spitsin SV, Kean RB, et al. Therapeutic intervention in experimental allergic encephalomyelitis by administration of uric acid precursors. *Proc Natl Acad Sci* 2002; 99:16303–16308.

Dietary Supplements: Cranberry and Other Supplements Used for Urinary Tract Infections

- Castello T, Girona L, Gomez MR, et al. The possible value of ascorbic acid as a prophylactic agent for urinary tract infection. *Spinal Cord* 1996; 34:592–593.

- Jellin JM, Gregory PJ, Batz F, et al. *Pharmacist's Letter/ Prescriber's Letter Natural Medicines Comprehensive*

Database. 4th ed. Stockton, CA: Therapeutic Research Faculty, 2002:421–422, 1259–1261, 1280–1286.

- Linsenmeyer T, Harrison B, Oakley A, et al. Evaluation of cranberry supplement for reduction of urinary tract infections in individuals with neurogenic bladders secondary to spinal cord injury. A prospective, double-blinded, placebo-controlled, crossover study. *J Spinal Cord Med* 2004; 27:29–34.

- Raz R, Chazan B, Dan M. Cranberry juice and urinary tract infection. *Clin Inf Dis* 2004; 38:1413–1419.

- Suvarna R. Possible interaction between warfarin and cranberry juice. *Brit Med J* 2003; 327:1454.

- Waites KB, Canupp KC, Armstrong S, et al. Effect of cranberry extract on bacteriuria and pyuria in persons with neurogenic bladder secondary to spinal cord injury. *J Spinal Cord Med* 2004; 27:35–40.

Dietary Supplements: Echinacea and Other "Immune-Stimulating" Supplements

- Bowling AC. *Alternative Medicine and Multiple Sclerosis*. New York: Demos Medical Publishing, 2001:106–107, 118–119, 183–206.

- Bowling AC, Ibrahim R, Stewart TM. Alternative medicine and multiple sclerosis: An objective review from an American perspective. *Int J MS Care* 2000; 2:14–21.

- Fetrow CW, Avila JR. *Professional's Handbook of Complementary & Alternative Medicines*. 2nd ed. Springhouse, PA: Springhouse Corp, 2001:275–278.

- Jellin JM, Gregory PJ, Batz F, et al. *Pharmacist's Letter/ Prescriber's Letter Natural Medicines Comprehensive Database*. 4th ed. Stockton, CA: Therapeutic Research Faculty, 2002:477–480.

- Schwarz S, Knauth M, Schwab S, et al. Acute disseminated encephalomyelitis after parenteral therapy with herbal extracts: a report of two cases. *J Neurol Neurosurg Psych* 2000; 69:516–518.

Dietary Supplements: Ginkgo Biloba

- Bowling AC. *Alternative Medicine and Multiple Sclerosis.* New York: Demos Medical Publishing, 2001: 108–109.

- Brochet B, Guinot P, Orgogozo J, et al. Double-blind, placebo controlled, multicentre study of ginkgolide B in treatment of acute exacerbations for multiple sclerosis. The Ginkgolide Study Group in multiple sclerosis. *J Neurol Neurosurg Psych* 1995; 58:360–362.

- Jellin JM, Gregory PJ, Batz F, et al. *Pharmacist's Letter/ Prescriber's Letter Natural Medicines Comprehensive Database.* 4th ed. Stockton, CA: Therapeutic Research Faculty, 2002:586–590.

- Kenney C, Norman, M, Jacobson M, et al. A double-blind, placebo-controlled, modified crossover pilot study of the effects of ginkgo biloba on cognitive and functional abilities in multiple sclerosis. *Neurol* 2002; 58: A458–A459.

Dietary Supplements: Kava Kava

- Clouatre DL. Kava kava: Examining new reports of toxicity. *Toxicol Lett* 2004; 150:85–96.

- Jellin JM, Gregory PJ, Batz F, et al. *Pharmacist's Letter/ Prescriber's Letter Natural Medicines Comprehensive Database.* 4th ed. Stockton, CA: Therapeutic Research Faculty, 2002:759–761.

- Mischoulon D, Rosenbaum JF. *Natural Medications for Psychiatric Disorders: Considering the Alternatives.* Philadelphia, PA: Lippincott Williams & Wilkins, 2002:128–129.

- Russo E. *Handbook of Psychotropic Herbs: A Scientific Analysis of Herbal Remedies for Psychiatric Conditions.* New York: Haworth Herbal Press, 2001:160–179.

Dietary Supplements: Padma 28

- Badnaev V, Kozlowski P, Schuller-Levis G, et al. The therapeutic effect of an herbal formula badmaev 28 (padma 28) on experimental allergic encephalomyelitis (EAE) in SJL/J mice. *Phytother Res* 1999; 13:218–221.

- Bowling AC, Stewart TM. Current complementary and alternative therapies for multiple sclerosis. *Curr Treat Options Neurol* 2003; 5:55–68.

- Korwin-Piotrowska T, Nocoñ, Stañkowska-Chomicz A, et al. Experience of padma 28 in multiple sclerosis. *Phytother Res* 1992; 6:133–136.

Dietary Supplements: Psyllium

- Bowling AC. *Alternative Medicine and Multiple Sclerosis*. New York: Demos Medical Publishing, 2001: 112–113.

- Fetrow CW, Avila JR. *Professional's Handbook of Complementary & Alternative Medicines*. 2nd ed. Springhouse, PA: Springhouse Corp, 2001:610–615.

- Jellin JM, Gregory PJ, Batz F, et al. *Pharmacist's Letter/ Prescriber's Letter Natural Medicines Comprehensive Database*. 4th ed. Stockton, CA: Therapeutic Research Faculty, 2002:175–177, 192–194.

Dietary Supplements: St. John's Wort

- Bowling AC. *Alternative Medicine and Multiple Sclerosis*. New York: Demos Medical Publishing, 2001: 113–115.

- Izzo AA. Drug interactions with St. John's wort (Hypericum perforatum): Review of the clinical evidence. *Int J Clin Pharmacol Ther* 2004; 42:139–148.

- Jellin JM, Gregory PJ, Batz F, et al. *Pharmacist's Letter/ Prescriber's Letter Natural Medicines Comprehensive*

Database. 4th ed. Stockton, CA: Therapeutic Research Faculty, 2002:1180–1184.

- Mischoulon D, Rosenbaum JF. *Natural Medications for Psychiatric Disorders: Considering the Alternatives.* Philadelphia, PA: Lippincott Williams & Wilkins, 2002:3–12.

- Werneke U, Horn O, Taylor DM. How effective is St. John's wort? The evidence revisited. *J Clin Psych* 2004; 65:611–617.

Dietary Supplements: Valerian

- Bowling AC. *Alternative Medicine and Multiple Sclerosis.* New York: Demos Medical Publishing, 2001: 116–117.

- Jellin JM, Gregory PJ, Batz F, et al. *Pharmacist's Letter/ Prescriber's Letter Natural Medicines Comprehensive Database.* 4th ed. Stockton, CA: Therapeutic Research Faculty, 2002:1262–1264.

- Mischoulon D, Rosenbaum JF. *Natural Medications for Psychiatric Disorders: Considering the Alternatives.* Philadelphia, PA: Lippincott Williams & Wilkins, 2002:132–146.

- Russo E. *Handbook of Psychotropic Herbs: A Scientific Analysis of Herbal Remedies for Psychiatric Conditions.* New York: The Haworth Herbal Press, 2001:95–106.

Dietary Supplements: Vitamin B$_{12}$

- Bowling AC, Stewart TM. Current complementary and alternative therapies for multiple sclerosis. *Curr Treat Options Neurol* 2003; 5:55–68.

- Goodkin D, Jacobsen D, Galvez N, et al. Serum cobalamin deficiency is uncommon in multiple sclerosis. *Arch Neurol* 1994; 51:1110–1114.

- Kira J, Tobimatus S, Goto I. Vitamin B_{12} metabolism and massive-dose methyl vitamin B_{12} therapy in Japanese patients with multiple sclerosis. *Int Med* 1994; 33:82–86.

- Loder C, Allawi J, Horrobin DF. Treatment of multiple sclerosis with lofepramine, L-phenylalanine, and vitamin B_{12}: mechanism of action and clinical importance: roles of the locus coeruleus and central noradrenergic systems. *Med Hyp* 2002; 59:594–602.

- Wade DT, Young CA, Chaudhuri KR, Davidson DLW. A randomized placebo controlled exploratory study of vitamin B_{12}, lofepramine, and L-phenylalanine (the "Cari Loder regime") in the treatment of multiple sclerosis. *J Neurol Neurosurg Psych* 2002; 73:246–249.

Dietary Supplements: Vitamin D and Calcium

- Cantorna M, Hayes C, DeLuca H. 1, 25-dihydroxyvitamin D3 reversibly blocks the progression of relapsing encephalomyelitis, a model of multiple sclerosis. *Proc Natl Acad Sci USA* 1996; 93:7861–7864.

- Cantorna M, Humpal-Winter J, DeLuca H. In vivo upregulation of interleukin-4 is one mechanism underlying the immunoregulatory effects of 1,25-dihydroxyvitamin D3. *Arch Biochem Biophys* 2000; 377:135–138.

- Fleming J, Hummel A, Beinlich B, et al. Vitamin D treatment of relapsing-remitting multiple sclerosis (RRMS): a MRI-based pilot study. *Neurol* 2000; 54:A338.

- Munger KL, Zhang SM, O'Reilly E, et al. Vitamin D intake and incidence of multiple sclerosis. *Neurol* 2004; 62:60–65.

- Smeltzer S, Zimmerman V, Capriotti T, et al. Osteoporosis risk factors and bone mineral density in women with MS. *Int J MS Care* 2000; 4:17–23, 29.

Dietary Supplements: Zinc

- Kumar N, Gross JB, Ahlskog JE. Copper deficiency myelopathy produces a clinical picture like subacute combined degeneration. *Neurol* 2004, 63:33–39.

- Prodan CI, Holland NR, Wisdom PJ, et al. CNS demyelination associated with copper deficiency and hyperzincemia. *Neurol* 2002, 59:1453–1456.

- Schiffer RB, Herndon RM, Eskin T. Effects of altered dietary trace metals upon experimental allergic encephalomyelitis. *NeuroToxicol* 1990; 11:443–450.

- Schiffer RB, McDermott MP, Copley C. A multiple sclerosis cluster associated with a small, north-central Illinois community. *Arch Environ Health* 2001; 56:389–395.

- Stein EC, Schiffer RB, Hall WJ, et al. Multiple sclerosis and the workplace: Report of an industry-based cluster. *Neurol* 1987; 37:1672–1677.

Diets: The Swank Diet

- Bowling AC. *Alternative Medicine and Multiple Sclerosis*. New York: Demos Medical Publishing, 2001:74–90.

- Bowling AC, Stewart TM. Current complementary and alternative therapies for multiple sclerosis. *Curr Treat Options Neurol* 2003; 5:55–68.

- Swank RL. Multiple sclerosis: Twenty years on low fat diet. *Arch Neurol* 1970; 23:460–74.

- Swank RL, Dugan BB. Effect of low saturated fat diet in early and late cases of multiple sclerosis. *Lancet* 1990; 336:37–9.

- Swank RL, Goodwin J. Review of MS patient survival on a Swank low saturated fat diet. *Nutr* 2003; 19:161–162.

Diets: Supplementation with Omega-6 Fatty Acids

- Bates D, Fawcett P, Shaw D, et al. Polyunsaturated fatty acids in treatment of acute remitting multiple sclerosis. *Brit Med J* 1978; 2:1390–1391.

- Bowling AC, Stewart TM. Current complementary and alternative therapies for multiple sclerosis. *Curr Treat Options Neurol* 2003; 5:55–68.

- Dworkin R, Bates D, Millar J, et al. Linoleic acid and multiple sclerosis: A reanalysis of three double-blind trials. *Neurol* 1984; 34:1441–1445.

- Millar J, Zilkha K, Langman M, et al. Double-blind trial of linoleate supplementation of the diet in multiple sclerosis. *Brit Med J* 1973; 1:765–768.

- Paty D. Double-blind trial of linoleic acid in multiple sclerosis. *Arch Neurol* 1983; 40:693–694.

Diets: Supplementation with Omega-3 Fatty Acids

- Bates D, Cartlidge N, French J, et al. A double-blind controlled trial of long chain n-3 polyunsaturated fatty acids in the treatment of multiple sclerosis. *J Neurol Neurosurg Psych* 1989, 52:18–22.

- Bowling AC, Stewart TM. Current complementary and alternative therapies for multiple sclerosis. *Curr Treat Options Neurol* 2003; 5:55–68.

- Goldberg P, Fleming M, Picard H. Multiple sclerosis: Decreased relapse rate through dietary supplementation with calcium, magnesium and vitamin D. *Med Hyp* 1986; 21:193–200.

- Nordvik I, Myhr K-M, Nyland H, et al. Effect of dietary advice and n-3 supplementation in newly diagnosed MS patients. *Acta Neurol Scand* 2000; 102:143–149.

- Weinstock-Guttman B, Baier M, Park Y, et al. Low fat dietary intervention with omega-3 fatty acid supplementation in multiple sclerosis patients. *Prostaglandins Leukotrienes Essential Fatty Acids* 2005; 73:392–404.

Feldenkrais

- Bowling AC. *Alternative Medicine and Multiple Sclerosis.* New York: Demos Medical Publishing, 2001:98–99.

- Johnson SK, Frederick J, Kaufman M, et al. A controlled investigation of bodywork in multiple sclerosis. *J Alt Complim Med* 1999; 5:237–43.

Guided Imagery and Relaxation

- Bowling AC. *Alternative Medicine and Multiple Sclerosis*. New York: Demos Medical Publishing, 2001: 135–139.

- Ernst E (ed.). *The Desktop Guide to Complementary and Alternative Medicine*. London: Mosby, 2001:69–72.

- Maguire BL. The effects of imagery on attitudes and moods in multiple sclerosis patients. *Alt Therapies* 1996; 2:75–9.

- Van Fleet S. Relaxation and imagery for symptom management: Improving patient assessment and individualizing treatment. *Oncol Nurs Forum* 2000; 27:501–510.

Hyperbaric Oxygen

- Bennett M, Heard R. Hyperbaric oxygen therapy for multiple sclerosis. *Cochrane Database Syst Rev* 2004; (1):CD003057.

- Bowling AC. *Alternative Medicine and Multiple Sclerosis*. New York: Demos Medical Publishing, 2001: 133–134.

- Fischer BH, Marks M, Reich T. Hyperbaric oxygen treatment of multiple sclerosis. A randomized, placebo-controlled, double-blind study. *New Eng J Med* 1983; 308:181–6.

- Kleijnen J, Knipschild P. Hyberbaric oxygen for multiple sclerosis: Review of controlled trials. *Acta Neurol Scand* 1995; 91:330–4.

Magnetic Field Therapy

- Bowling AC. *Alternative Medicine and Multiple Sclerosis*. New York: Demos Medical Publishing, 2001: 140–143.

- Guseo A. Pulsing electromagnetic field therapy of multiple sclerosis by the Gyuling-Bordács device: Double-blind, cross-over and open studies. *J Bioelec* 1987; 6:23–35.

- Lappin MS, Lawrie FW, Richards TL, et al. Effects of a pulsed electromagnetic therapy on multiple sclerosis fatigue and quality of life: A double-blind, placebo controlled trial. *Alt Therap* 2003; 9:38–48.

- Nielsen JF, Sinkjaer T, Jakobsen J. Treatment of spasticity with repetitive magnetic stimulation; A double-blind placebo-controlled study. *Mult Scler* 1996; 2:227–32.

- Richards TL, Lappin MS, Acosta-Urquidi J, et al. Double-blind study of pulsing magnetic field effects on multiple sclerosis. *J Alt Complem Med* 1997; 3:21–9.

Massage

- Bowling AC. *Alternative Medicine and Multiple Sclerosis.* New York: Demos Medical Publishing, 2001: 148–151.

- Hernandez-Reif M, Field T, Field T, et al. Multiple sclerosis patients benefit from massage therapy. *J Bodywork Movement Ther* 1998; 2:168–74.

- Vickers A, *Massage and Aromatherapy: A Guide for Health Professionals.* London: Chapman & Hall, 1996.

Neural Therapy

- Gibson RG, Gibson SLM. Neural therapy in the treatment of multiple sclerosis. *J Altern Compl Med* 1999; 5:543–552.

Reflexology

- Bowling AC. *Alternative Medicine and Multiple Sclerosis.* New York: Demos Medical Publishing, 2001: 171–172.

- Siev-Nur I, Gamus D, Lerner-Geva L, Achiron A. Reflexology treatment relieves symptoms of multiple sclerosis: A randomized controlled study. *Mult Scler* 2003; 9:356–361.

Tai Chi

- Bowling AC. *Alternative Medicine and Multiple Sclerosis.* New York: Demos Medical Publishing, 2001: 173–175.

- Husted C, Pham L, Hekking A, et al. Improving quality of life for people with chronic conditions: The example of t'ai chi and multiple sclerosis. *Altern Ther* 1999; 5:70–4.

- Mills M, Allen J. Mindfulness of movement as a coping strategy in multiple sclerosis. A pilot study. *Gen Hosp Psych* 2000; 22:425–431.

- Wang C, Collet JP, Lau J. The effect of tai chi on health outcomes in patients with chronic conditions: A systematic review. *Arch Int Med* 2004; 164:493–501.

Yoga

- Bowling AC. *Alternative Medicine and Multiple Sclerosis.* New York: Demos Medical Publishing, 2001: 207–209.

- Depres L. Yoga and MS. *Yoga J* 1997; July/August: 96–103.

- Oken BS, Kishiyama S, Zajdel D, et al. Randomized controlled trial of yoga and exercise in multiple sclerosis. *Neurol* 2004; 62:2058–2064.

Index

5 - 10/08